Diets That Work

Weight-loss programmes Reviewed

Anne Alexander

Diets That Work

Copyright © 2017 Diets That Work

ISBN 978-1-900401-16-6

Also available as an e-Book / Kindle
ISBN 978-1-900401-15-9

     www.DietsThatWork.co.uk

Diets that Work

This book is dedicated to

those who are struggling with their weight.

May you now get as slim as you wish

And feel a million times better

CONTENTS

The book is divided into three distinct sections. The first (Section A – FOODS) covers the various types of food plus particular foods. The second section (B – SUPPLEMENTS) covers food additives or supplements available and the third section (C- DIETS) is about the various systems and diet programmes that we have found work best and fastest. Finally, at the back of the book (D- APPENDICES) are some references chapters covering additional items that may assist.

Diets That Work

INTRODUCTION
An independent review of weight-loss systems

I've written this book as an independent review of various weight-loss diets that I've tried and evaluated either personally or my friends and acquaintances have. The book covers those diet systems that we're sure can help you lose weight, safely; your health and well-being are one of your most important assets!

Everyone strives to get to an optimum weight but its not easy with so many delicious foods (and drinks!). I've tried many methods and countless diet systems to lose weight; some have worked, but some sadly have not and seem to be a waste of time (and money!). There is a wealth of information on diets, but unfortunately some of it is very confusing and it's very easy to develop a case of 'information overload'.

I've been asked by many friends to share some of the diets that have been found to work. It's an honour to share with you some of the diets that my friends and I know work.

Even modest weight loss, perhaps around 5 to 10%, can make a huge difference to your body and it can significantly improve your health. Such a modest loss could easily prevent you succumbing to some debilitating diseases. It could also save you a lot of time (and money too). There's no better or more reliable proof than first hand experience of a product; that's what I offer in this book and on my web site (http://Diets That Work.co.uk).

Hopefully some diets will work for you too? Please do let us know your comments and your experiences, and whether you find these pages useful.

The web pages have been designed to be easy to digest (no pun intended!) and to have all the information and links you will need. The site is updated and revised frequently.

Diets that Work

Anyone can lose weight - it's easy!

The hardest bit of any diet is maintenance, or keeping weight off. Less than 2% of those on diets succeed in keeping the weight down. It's so easy to pile it on again. Even modest weight loss, perhaps around 5 to 10%, can make a huge difference to your body and it can significantly improve your health. More importantly, such a modest loss could easily prevent you succumbing to some debilitating diseases.

In this book I've looked at several different aspects of food consumption and ways of dieting. Included are many tips and summaries of my findings. The website and the e-book also have hypertext links to many of the books, courses, videos and other help that were useful and that my team and I thought might also help you. The reviews of diet products, books or equipment are all written by myself or parts by my friends independently; we did not accept any gifts or assistance from the suppliers of any products in connection with this book.

I am not a dietician or qualified as a nutritionist. I sought professional help in compiling this guide and to qualify as a 'Diet that Works', I saw the effect on myself or a close friend or acquaintance. I have left out of the book any mentions of products which we found had unfortunate side-effects.

During the diet assessments I didn't do any strenuous exercise or use professional equipment. Some trainers maintain that you can only lose weight by strenuous exercise, so I have included some information about training equipment, at the back of the book.

I hope you enjoy reading the book and find information in your search for a slimmer you, while making your body healthy. Please feel free to contact me with your comments, I really would love to hear from YOU.

Wishing you successful slimming

Anne Alexander

E-Mail anne@dietsthatwork.co.uk

You are what you eat

And if you enjoy your food
You will enjoy your body too!

A   FOODS

Types of Foods

Almost all of the many kinds of foods we eat can be simply categorised into one of just five types:

- Animal Products

- Fats and Oils

- Fruits

- Grains

- Seeds

We also consume an ever increasingly wide variety of manufactured ingredients; these are mostly replacements for naturally occurring foodstuffs. Generally speaking, it is more healthy to try to avoid artificially manufactured ingredients and processed foods. It's much better to stick with whole, nutrient-rich foods instead.

The nutrients found in foods are also in one of five categories:

- Anti-nutrients (e.g. phytic & oxalic acid)

- Fat and fatty Acids

- Vitamins

- Protein

- Fibre

Calories

Calories are a measure of energy, normally used to measure the energy content of foods and beverages.

Technically speaking, a dietary calorie is a scientific unit that can be measured accurately. It is defined as the amount of energy required to raise the temperature of 1 kilogram of water by 1 degree Celsius.

Our bodies use the calories in the food that we eat and drink for essential functions such as breathing and thinking, as well as day-to-day activities such as walking, talking and eating.

On average a man will use about 2,500 calories a day and a woman 1500 calories a day just to keep their metabolism ticking over. If they get out of bed and do something, their body will burn up more than that.

Everyone's weight, and the amount and rate it is gained and lost, depends on the amount of calories they consume and burn up. As you might expect, bodies lose weight when less calories are consumed than the body uses.

Conversely, a body will increase in weight when more calories are eaten than are expended. As an approximation, to lose one pound of fat, a body needs to use up around 3,500 calories. This can be done either through exercise or diet.

Imagine someone weighing 14 or 15 stones wanting to lose one pound in a week. Through the use of an exercise regime alone, they will needs to run about 3.5 miles per day. A total of 24.5 miles over the week. This assumes that their diet remains the same. If that person relies solely on dieting, they would need to reduce their intake by at least 500 calories each day, assuming that their exercise regime remains the same.

Diets that Work

Calorie Counting
It can make or break your diet

Calorie counters and nutrient trackers are incredibly useful if you are trying to lose, maintain or even gain weight. They can also help if you are trying to make specific changes to your diet, such as eating such as varying the proportions of protein or carbs that you eat.

There is no need for most people to track their intake all the time; its far better to do it just every now and then to get a general picture of what you are eating.

Do calories count?

You often hear people claim that calories don't matter and calorie counting is a waste of time. However, when it comes to your weight, calories most certainly DO count.

This is a fact that has been proven time and time again in scientific experiments called overfeeding studies.

The studies on the Authority Nutrition website prove this. These studies asked the subjects to deliberately overeat and subsequently they measured the impact on their weight and health.

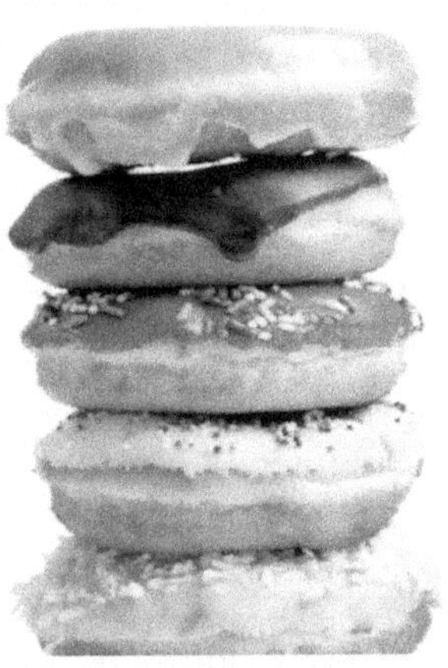

All overfeeding studies have found that, when people eat more calories than they burn off each day, they **gain weight.**

Diets That Work

Importance of Diet   QUALITY & QUANTITY
Calories are useful for keeping tabs on the quantity of food that we consume, but they don't measure the QUALITY of the food, or of the drink.

However, it's important to note that, when it comes to foods and the human body, then a calorie is not necessarily a calorie! One hundred calories of healthy and natural vegetables will have a very different effect on your health than will rather 100 calories of chips or crisps, or a sugary doughnut.

The way the body processes calories varies enormously. Some will be turned into fat, which is then deposited in places where you would rather not have it, while some calories will be turned into energy, burning away some existing fat. Other food will be processed into cellular tissue, muscles and so on, and some will add very little at all and just be processed through the digestive system.

The types of foods that you eat have a huge effect on your health, so the composition of your diet is of considerable importance.

Different types of food have varying effects on hunger, appetite hormones and so the amount of calories that your body can burn from these can vary considerably. A diet that is based on high-quality foods, such as those from plants or animals that have been minimally processed, is going to have more effect on weight loss.

Exercise does not make much difference
Weight loss measured by calorie expenditure through exercise, is relatively small in the grand scheme of things. Most of the calories that we use are burned up just "staying alive." The calories burned in this way is known as our "resting metabolic rate." An average size man burns over 2,000 calories a day with no physical exertion. It takes a huge amount of additional exercise to make much of a difference to their calorific burn rate.

Diets that Work

Some people contend that carbohydrates and insulin are the main problems controlling weight loss and weight gain. This is known as "the insulin hypothesis of obesity." While the control of insulin and carbohydrates and insulin may have some important for some people, the hypothesis in general has proven flawed.

Carbs & Calorie Counter
by Chris Ceyett

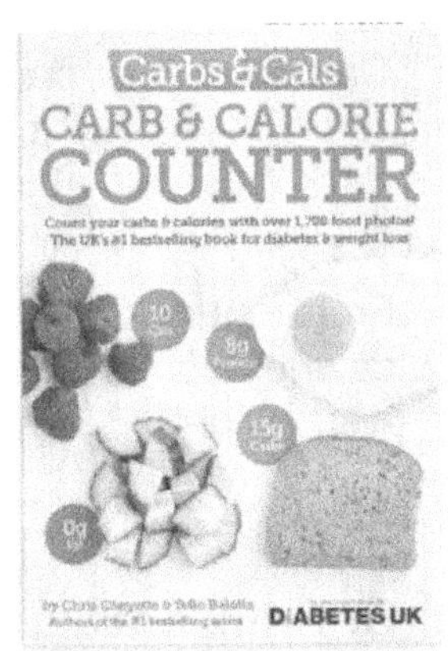

Now you can count both your carbs and calories with over 1700 photos of food and drink. This is a 352 page book, sent to you immediately and with FREE P&P.

Recognised all over the English speaking world as THE "Carb & Calorie counting bible". It has a unique visual method of showing hundreds of food photos that makes counting carbs and calories so simple and straight forward. Each food item has up to 6 portion photos, so it's a breeze to choose the right portions and make weight control easier.

This is a great resource for managing diabetes, a weight loss programme, portion control and or just general healthy eating.

* Over 1,700 food & drink photos
* Nutrients in colour-coded circles

* Values for carbs, calories, protein, fat, and fibre

* Introduction on healthy eating,

* The latest nutritional values

* Tables showing nutritional values

Diets That Work

Authority Nutrition is an independent organisation that provides daily articles about nutrition, weight loss and health. All their statements are based on scientific evidence, and are written only by experts with a deep knowledge of nutrition. Their website is completely unbiased, and 100% independent.

The Authority Nutrition are not sponsored by any industry or company.

On one of their pages they have a simple but highly accurate scientific calorie calculator, which we have found helps to track calorie intake and thus weight. There are five evidence-based tips on how to sustainably reduce calorie intake.

From your details entered into the calculator it will suggest calories you should be eating each day to either maintain or lose weight.

Dr Briffa's Weight Studies

In his health blog, **Dr. John Briffa,** analysed a study examining weight loss without dietary intervention.

In this study, 320 post-menopausal women whose weight ranged from normal to obese were taken at random to either an additional exercise or no additional exercise group (the control group).

Those in the exercise group were instructed to take 45 minutes worth of moderate to vigorous aerobic exercise, 5 times a week for a year. Both groups (the additional exercise and the control group) were instructed not to change their diets.

At the end of the first year, Dr Briffa found that the exercise group, compared to the control group, lost an average of 2 kilograms (4.4 pounds) of fat.

If you are one of those who would like to lose that amount of fat, you may be interested to hear what those ladies had to accomplish in terms of exercise to lose that much fat?

Diets that Work

Foods you can eat lots of and stay THIN

1. Pears and apples
These delicious superfruits are loaded with antioxidants and are good for you for many reasons. They also are loaded with fibre. They cut your appetite and make you feel full.

2. Lentils and beans
Just one serving of lentils gives you 11 grams of fiber and 13 grams of protein. These and other legumes make you feel 31% more full when compared to foods like bread and pasta. One study said that eating beans is more satisfying than eating beef.

3. Greek yogurt and cottage cheese
Dairy foods of all types are very good at keeping you feeling full. It may help to limit dairy for a number of reasons but Greek yogurt and cottage cheese should always be in your fridge.

One recent study showed that people who ate a high protein Greek yogurt as a snack after lunch were less hungry later than those who ate lower protein yogurt.

4. Eggs
Eating two eggs gives you 12 grams of complete protein and loads of essential amino acids that your body needs. One study showed that people who ate eggs at breakfast had stable blood sugar levels and felt less hungry for a full day after, one of the key requirements of maintaining low weight.

5. Beef
Just 4 ounces of lean beef has 32 grams of protein and plenty of amino acids. Just make sure you know how to shop for healthy beef. You don't want to eat too much of it, but when you do it's sure to keep you feeling full.

6. Broth-based soups
Soups that are broth based are high in both protein and water. Those 2 things together combine to make you feel full. A pot of soup loaded with vegetables, lentils, or chicken can keep you feeling full for a long time. If you need some good

Diets That Work

soup recipes, there are FIVE excellent ones by Danette May on the soups page of our web site.

7. Hot Oatmeal

Studies say that part of the magic is in the warmth of the meal. This is because when you heat up oatmeal in coconut or almond milk, it has a higher level of thickness, and that makes you feel full.

8. Avocado

Avocado is a perfect example of a plant-based fat that will keep you feeling full. One study showed that half of an avocado increased satisfaction by 26% and reduced hunger by 40% for 3 hours.

9. Jackfruit

A delicious, sweet, juicy fruit when it is ripe, the jackfruits are also seen as one of the newest, hottest meat substitutes. They are often eaten by both vegans and vegetarians, and seem to be at their most nutritious before they ripen.

10. Quinoa

Quinoa is a complete protein that has TWICE the fibre of brown rice. It will suppress hunger for a long time while providing lots of great nutrition.

An excellent way to enjoy quinoa is in Danette May's *Zesty Mexican Quinoa Skillet or as a Quinoa Chilli,* as described on our web site. You'll love how easy this delicious one pan recipe is to throw together.

11. Coconut

These nuts are full of natural goodness and their oil has even more excellent properties. Read more about coconut, its oil and their advantages on the *Diets That Work* web site, where you can get a copy of the fascinating report about the benefits it can have on your thyroid by Susan Patterson.

Organic Foods

The term 'organic' means a wholly natural product grown without the help of chemical or synthetic pesticides, antibiotics, growth stimulants or unnatural insecticides.

All organic food is supposed to be fully traceable from farm to fork, so that you are able to be sure of what you're eating. The standards for organic food are laid down in European law so any food labeled as organic must meet strict rules.

Organic food is produced on organic farms using a more natural but strictly controlled system of farm management. Unlike non-organic food production, which uses manufactured and mined fertilisers and pesticides, organic food is produced and grown using natural fertilization product made from plants. Organic food is usually produced using less energy and with more respect for the animals that provide it.

Organic farming and food production is not always the easiest way of doing it and takes real commitment and attention to detail. The work is invariably backed up by rigorous, independent inspection and certification.

Organic Foods

While many fruit and vegetable can be eaten without adding too much weight, the ten most common ones that you can eat a lot of without putting on too much weight are listed below:

If a food is made with 70% organic ingredients it is allowed to state "made with organic ingredients" on the label.

Turmeric

Turmeric dry root extract and dry leaf of artichoke extract can aid digestion and help maintain a healthy bowel. Turmeric's powers have been well known for couple of millennia, the ancient Greeks and the Egyptians were (and still are) big users of Turmeric.

Diets That Work

Among the many advantages of Turmeric are:

Helps Protect Brain Cells

Turmeric binds to and dissolves abnormal proteins in the brain, helping to protect them from damage. It reduces one of the main factors of memory loss - brain plaque.

Helps Maintain a Healthy Inflammatory Response

Studies confirm that Turmeric is one of the most powerful antioxidants. It can free radicals and may reduce or even prevent some of the damage they cause. Turmeric lowers the levels of two enzymes in the body that cause inflammation.

Supports healthy Cardiovascular Function

It may support your heart by saving it from the damaging effects of chronic inflammation. Because it stops platelets from clumping together, turmeric may also prevent blood clots from building up along the walls of arteries.

Helps maintain a Positive Attitude

Studies show many noticeable and promising results with turmeric for supporting a balanced and positive mood.

Promotes Radiant Skin

Research shows that turmeric inhibits a key enzyme (*elastase*) that reduces the ability of elastin from forming. *Elastin*, and collagen are proteins that make the skin smooth and pliable.

Enhances Detoxification

Turmeric stimulates your liver helping detoxify from toxins, metals, heavy metals and other toxins clogging up your system.

 www.DietsThatWork.co.uk

Diets that Work

Turmeric is a wonderful food product that has been in use for at least 4,000 years! One of the easiest ways to get and store it ready for use is as Purathrive's **Lipolife Turmeric.** I found it to be a very useful product and suggest that you get some NOW.

Liposomal Curcumin

Liposomal's turmeric and curcumin technology protects the nutrient from being destroyed in your stomach and delivers the nutrient directly to your cells. In fact, "Data shows that Liposomal Delivery is up to 20 times more Bio-Available than Conventional Methods"

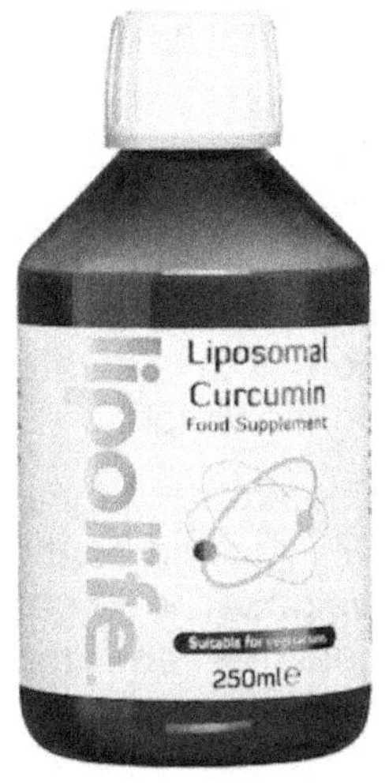

Most turmeric supplements are poorly absorbed by your body and you may be "peeing" them out with NO benefit. That's why we've talked with the most brilliant minds in science today and discovered something called "liposomes".

Liposomes are little protection systems designed to protect and deliver nutrients straight into the bloodstream. Liposomes were first discovered in breast milk to enhance delivery of key nutrients to babies.

They act as microscopic bodyguards, grabbing hold of and protecting nutrients (in this case, turmeric) as they travel through your digestive system, through your bloodstream and deliver it straight into your cells, completely undamaged.

Enzymes in the mouth and stomach, digestive juices, bile salts (to neutralize the digestive acids) and various flora in the intestines can break-down and degrade the supplement. You can find full details of the Liposomal Curcumin on the web site.

Diets That Work

Organic 7-Day Total Body Reset

This Ph.D verified course can help you drop body-fat and live a healthier, less painful, more active life in just 7 days. Celebrity trainer **Thomas Delauer** has appeared on many TV shows and on the front cover of such prestigious fitness and training magazines as *Muscle & Performance, Ironman* and *Icon.*

Our web site has a short video presentation and other information about this exciting new **7-Day Body Reset** system.

It's natural, organic and it certainly does make you lose weight. It will help fight the curse of inflammation, one of the things that may be hurting your body, sending your brain all the wrong signals. These signals are probably sending your body into 'starvation mode' and this could be making you pile on the weight.

The amazing thing is that this priceless information costs only $7 - it could be the best thing you do all year to help you lose weight. The Organic 7-day should be your passport to a far healthier and more active life using a simple but quite revolutionary seven day programme.

Coconut and its Oil

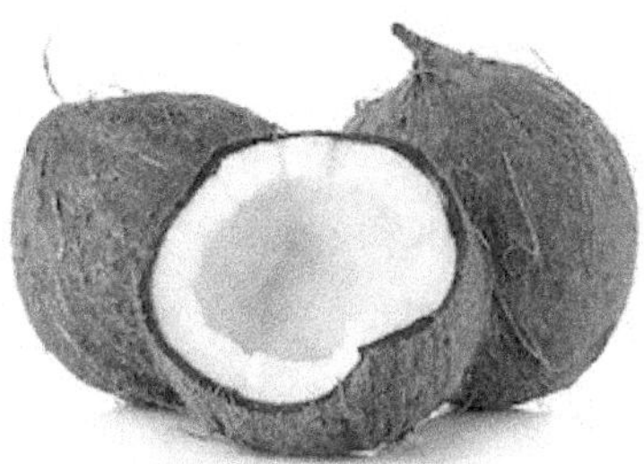

One of the cheapest yet the most wholesome product you can find. It is a member of the Arecaceae family and the only species of the genus called Cocos. The term coconut can refer to the whole coconut palm or the seed, or the fruit. The fruit is technically or botanically speaking not a nut at all, but a drupe!

Coconut is the main item in the diet of almost a third of the planet but in the UK and western Europe is regarded as an exotic fruit, mainly as they don't grow natively in northern Europe. It's got three layers: the exocarp or outside layer, the matty husk (called the mesocarp) which is inside it, and the nut fibre inside, often called the white 'meat' of the coconut.

Coconuts have been around for tens of thousands of years and for at least five thousand years have been used by mankind for fuel, building, food and even as musical instruments. One of the coconuts' biggest and most useful functions has been as a medicine. They can help to cure fevers, nausea, rashes, earache, sore throat, bronchitis, kidney stones, ulcers, asthma, syphilis, dropsy, toothache, bruises, and even body lice!

Diets That Work

Some common ailments that coconut helps cure:

- Coughs
- Constipation
- Malnutrition
- Skin Infections
- Toothaches
- Earaches
- Influenza

Coconut is one of nature's most versatile and powerful products that can bring huge improvements to many aspects of your life:

- Dental health (fights plaque, removes stains & makes your teeth whiter too!)
- Brain health – boosts activity
- Weight-loss
- Oral hygiene by detoxifying your mouth
- Reduces halitosis
- Gum health
- Digestive issues

Teeth Whitening can be scary and uncomfortable using chemicals - dangerous too. But all you really need is Coconut. *LiveCoco* have a range of coconut products that are a great alternative to the usual chemical products.

One excellent *Livecoco* product is their 100% Natural Teeth Whitening & Oral Detox solution. It uses Coconut Oil (known as Oil Pulling) and is 100% natural, gluten-free & vegan friendly. There is more information about *LiveCoCo Teeth Whitening & Oral Detox,* on our web site.

Diets that Work

COCONUT & the thyroid

There are many signs that your thyroid is not performing correctly; do you know how to spot them? Is it your weight? If you struggle to lose fat despite exercising and eating properly, or if you have low energy levels, difficulty sleeping, sensitivity to either extreme cold or to heat, if you suffer from digestive issues, or the dreaded 'brain fog' then it's possible that you might have a thyroid disorder.

It's estimated that up to 10% of people are afflicted by thyroid problems and it seems increasingly common that people are being found to have issues with or connected to their thyroid.

There are various ways in which you can detect if your thyroid is not functioning correctly. On our web site is a link to a FREE article by Susan Patterson which explains how you can simply test for thyroid malfunction. She also explains why so many thyroid medications are ineffective, and how you can feed your thyroid with the naturally occurring saturated fat in coconut oil, which has some amazing therapeutic properties.

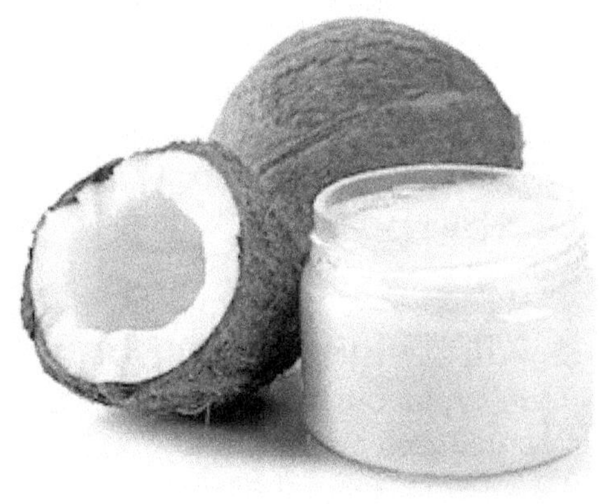

COCONUT OILS

No man-made food product concocted in a laboratory has yet managed to replace the value of what is found in nature!

Mother Nature is incredibly generous with the abundance of healthy nutritious food she provides. A bounty of fruits and vegetables rich in vitamins, minerals and nutrients to nourish your body so you can enjoy a long healthy life

One fruit in particular - the coconut - is so abundant in its healing properties it's often referred to by many as "the tree of life." Before World War II, people living in island countries, like the Philippines, the Caribbean Islands or places like Hawaii, lived on a diet that consisted mainly of rice, root crops, vegetables and huge amounts of the ultra-healing 'super food', the coconut.

The coconut is a "functional food" rich in vitamins, minerals and fiber - the essential nutritional building blocks for perfect health.

It's excellent as a sun tan lotion, as a shampoo, as a skin conditioner and also it is said to stop hair turning grey. Many say it has cancer-inhibiting properties, but that's yet to be proven, but it certainly is an anti-oxidant.

Coconut helps weight loss.
Coconut based dishes as part of a structured diet can promote weight loss. With coconut oil as part of your diet, you are more likely to lose weight more quickly and more safely.

Coconuts KILL high Blood Sugar
In a study published by the *British Journal of Nutrition* in 2003, participants, both diabetic and non-diabetic, were given a variety of foods to eat. These foods included cinnamon bread, carrot cake, brownies, granola, and other foods that people with diabetes should normally carefully limit.

Diets that Work

When the study was conducted, it was found that when this FATTY food was increased, the blood sugar response between the two groups was nearly identical.

Not only healthy, it's delicious

The health report provides delicious recipes that you'll be craving after just one try! Healthy has never tasted so good! Start your day with a blueberry coconut smoothie! Talk about an antioxidant double-whammy!

Coconut stir-fried vegetables!

Makes vegetables taste delicious, you will be amazed!

Coconut chicken

One of our personal favorites! It is likely to soon become your family's favorite meal! And many more delicious recipes that would even make a master chef jealous!

These and many more delicious meals can be found in an eleven item recipe book which is part of the Coconut Triple Whammy Offer detailed below. The package contains all the information you need to turn out delicious healthy meals your body and family will love you for.

Coconut Books Triple Package

1. The Coconut Oil Secret

     (Natures best healing Superfood)

2. 20 Anti-aging & cleansing with Coconut Oil

3. 11 Healthy Recipes using Coconut Oil

are the three special reports available in a Triple Package of Coconut reports. You also get an exclusive guide that shares the secrets of the 'Tree of Life' that is coconut. All the details are on the 'Coconut' page on the *Diets That Work* web site.

Soups

Freshly made soup is not only much tastier than a dried or canned product, it is far better for you as it still contains all the healthy ingredients such as vitamins.

Processed soups however are a very different 'kettle of fish'. The canned and dried types will be largely processed and have the goodness already cooked out of them. They are little more than a filler, much of the content of the ingredients will add calories and weight. They will be filling, yes, but not such a great idea if you are trying to LOSE weight.

It's hard to go wrong with a good soup recipe! Soups offer the most tremendous versatility to your family's menus because they can be served as a starter but also work perfectly as a main dish.

Soups contain lots of water, which you need to clear the body of the toxins, and keep you hydrated. can be stored in the freezer for quick "heat and eat" meals that can be quickly taken while "on the run."

There are plenty of great soup recipes around, there are five on the soups page in the FOOD section of the Diets That Work web site. The page has five delicious recipes from a leading American nutritionist, **Danette May,** that will warm your belly and soothe your soul! They are very nutritious and will help you shed those pounds.

Danette's recipes have gone down very well in our house and are already having great effect. (Some of Danette's training can be found in a chapter about her diet regime in Section C, further on in this book and on our web site).

Diets that Work

Desserts

Can you have Chocolate Cake on a diet?

Absolutely!

e.g. Chocolate Cake

Key Lime Pie

Lemon Meringe

There are tremendous recipes for some of the mouth-watering desserts that we can now enjoy without feeling guilty or piling on the pounds. Some of the recipes have been devised by well-known trainers such as Kelsey Ale, Adriana Harlan or Danette May.

The desserts suggested on the *Diets That Work* web site taste even BETTER than they look. They are all made from natural ingredients and so can help you lose weight.

The desserts that we have found ARE suitable for weight loss have all the goodness of a regular everyday cake, but they are in a much healthier Paleo version. That means they are loaded with fibre, vitamins, antioxidants, healthy fats, and minerals. They are all 100% gluten-free as they have no grain ingredients and are all much lower in sugar than 'normal' cakes, desserts and other confectionaries.

You can make a delicious chocolate cake with healthy ingredients like eggs, coconut oil, cocoa, honey, sea salt, stevia and wholesome dark chocolate. Normal chocolate cakes, especially those bought retail, are usually a disaster for your health. Loaded with hydrogenated oils, corn syrup solids, refined wheat flour, refined sugar and other ingredients that damage your body.

Diets That Work

Here are some other examples of tasty delicious desserts that Kelsey shows you how to make healthy versions of in her book: all these delicious paleo cakes are gluten-free, soy-free, no added refined sugar and they can be made dairy-free if you prefer!

Banana Bundt Cake

Flourless Fudge Brownie

Peach Melba Pie

Brownies

Pineapple Upside-Down Cake

Key Lime Pie

Salted Caramel Ice Cream

With these dessert menus you can have your favourite pie, flan or cake for any meal, even for breakfast!

In fact leading Australian nutritionist Nicole Joy has written couple of books telling you just how and what you can eat while still losing weight. Her successful *'Eat Desserts for Breakfast'* is hard to find in the stores, but you can get it by mail order and we strongly recommend you get a copy of it so you can begin enjoying desserts again! We know it will really enlighten you and show you all the yummy treats you have been missing out on if you have been on a strict diet. No more – the good days are ahead!

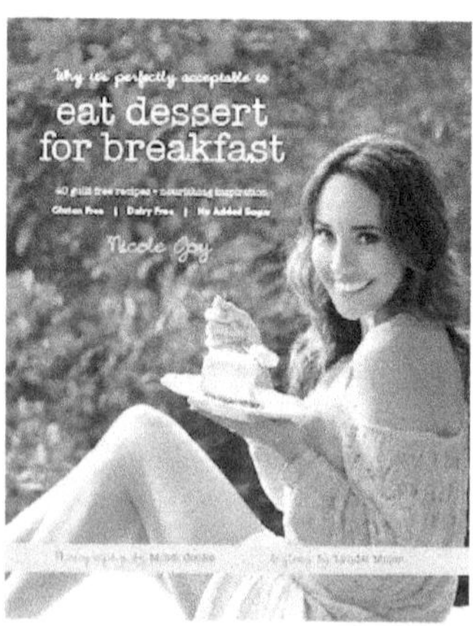

Diets that Work

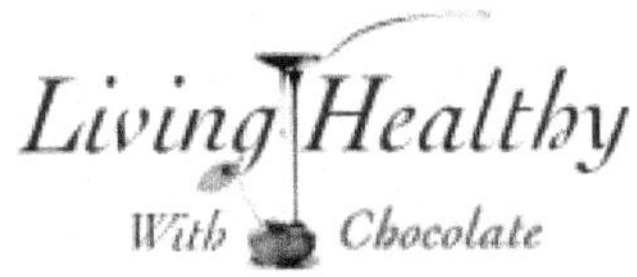

Living Healthy with Chocolate

Books that are genuinely about healthier eating are pretty rare, but Living Healthy with Chocolate is well worth telling you about. It's packed with ways you can make delicious desserts, a bit decadent, but actually they're GOOD FOR YOU.

Author **Adriana Harlan**, struggled with sugar cravings for years; by careful research in her own kitchen, she found the secret to maintaining her optimal weight and living without the effects of inflammation that troubles so many of us.

Adriana lives in Hawaii and is a self-confessed chocaholic. She worked for many years as an oceanographer. One of her favourite desserts is her '**Molten Lava Brownies**' which are paleo, gluten free and dairy free but still have what she describes as " an ooey, gooey centre that your just fall in love with."

Another of Adriana's favourites (and mine too!) is Strawberry Tuiles with fresh strawberries and chocolate whipped cream. Originally a French dessert, these cookies are crispy and shaped into either arcs or cones. You've probably had them before with other desserts. Adriana modified the recipe and substituted the flour and refined sugars. The result is a sweet, chewy cookie that tastes amazing!

She is passionate about healthy eating and loves developing new baking and cooking techniques. Recently she has been teaching people how to cook healthy food and in response to lots of requests she decided to write about it.

Living Healthy With Chocolate is the result and it can help YOU to turn out delicious desserts too, but by leaving out the dangerous things like gluten, refined sugar, processed foods and soy. They are replaced with natural and healthy ingredients.

Diets That Work

In her book, Adriana demonstrates how YOU can cook healthy meals and gorgeous desserts that look deliciously decadent. One of the delights of eating is in the appearance of food and there is little that looks more scrumptious than the texture of a nice gooey chocolate cake!

Adriana's desserts use nutrient-rich ingredients enabling YOU to have a more balanced, healthier and much happier life. Adriana's recipes don't contain ANY refined and processed ingredients. They don't contain the potentially dangerous ingredients like the dreaded refined sugars, which are what she found are what give us pangs of hunger and cravings for food that isn't always good for us.

Using her degree in biology she has dug deep into many scientific studies to arrive at her solutions of how to produce delicious chocolate desserts that are

Living Healthy with Chocolate isn't available in bookshops but you can get information through a link on the DESSERTS page of our web site.

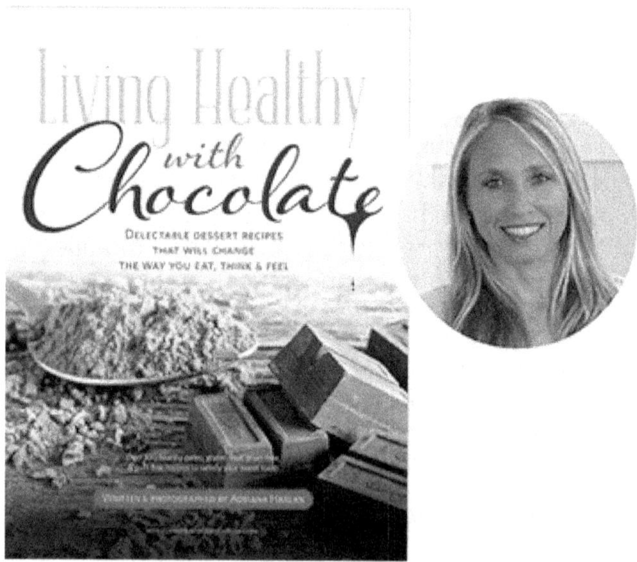

Diets that Work

Diabetes

A few hard truths about Diabetes

Countless studies from scientists and doctors all over the world have proven that people with 'Type 2 diabetes' can normalise blood sugar, increase insulin sensitivity, reduce neuropathy pain, lower risk of blindness, amputations and be taken off all diabetes drugs and insulin injections.

It might be hard to believe, but when you prick your finger with a meter and see a blood sugar reading of let's say 250, it's NOT because you have diabetes! Some people can walk around with blood sugar as high as 300 without having diabetes. How is this possible? Simple - INFLAMMATION.

Ever wondered why diabetics have such high rates of heart disease, heart attacks, cancer, high cholesterol, blindness, arthritis, and neuropathy? Inflammation. Just recently in February 2015, scientists and researchers at the University of California San Diego proved that 'Type 2' diabetes is caused by inflammation: they discovered that an inflammatory molecule called LTB4 causes insulin resistance.

And what does insulin resistance lead to? high blood sugar and diabetes. This is the reason why treating your blood sugar with drugs and injecting insulin to combat insulin sensitivity will never heal your diabetes; because you aren't treating the root cause of diabetes, just the symptoms of it.

Diets That Work

Reverse Your Type 2 Diabetes

Diabetics CAN take their health back into their own hands.

If you are diabetic, you CAN free yourself from the shackles of constant blood sugar readings, daily drug regimes and even prevent the horrible health complications that await diabetics further down the road of life.

There are hundreds of suppressed scientific studies and powerful medical research that have now been condensed into an easy to read and understand, step-by-step health guide called "***The 7 Steps to Health and the Big Diabetes Lie***".

It has already been used to help tens of thousands of diabetics all over the world. These are life changing scientifically proven diabetes treatment methods.

7 Steps to Health and the Big Diabetes Lie is available as an e-book or as a paperback; all the details about how you can get a copy of the book and maybe help someone special in your life to reverse their Type 2 diabetes, are on our web site on the Diabetes pages. The site also has some extracts from the book to read before you buy a copy of it. It comes with a money back guarantee too; sixty days to decide if it's for you, or your money back.

Sweeteners

This chapter deals with both natural and artificial sweeteners. In over 85% of the world, we have all been brought up to crave sweet tasting food. Its very hard to lose that conditioning, and it's a simple thing to address.

Some of the sweetest and tastiest sweeteners are not easily available. You may want to look into a couple of these:

Swanson's Lo Han Sweetener is a concentrated extract that is obtained from a traditional Chinese fruit. It's also grown in other countries where it's more commonly known as Monk Fruit.

It's now been refined and marketed in the west as an ideal way to sweeten drinks. It has no bitterness, like some other sweeteners, and is extremely low in calorific content. It reportedly has zero, or virtually no calories. Lo Han tastes around two hundred times sweeter than sugar, so you don't need very much of it (see other relative taste values of other sweeteners below).

The natural sweetness of the Swanson product has been tempered a little by blending it with natural inulin (an oligosaccharide that is digested by bacteria in the gut and converted into short chain triglycerides which help make T-cells).

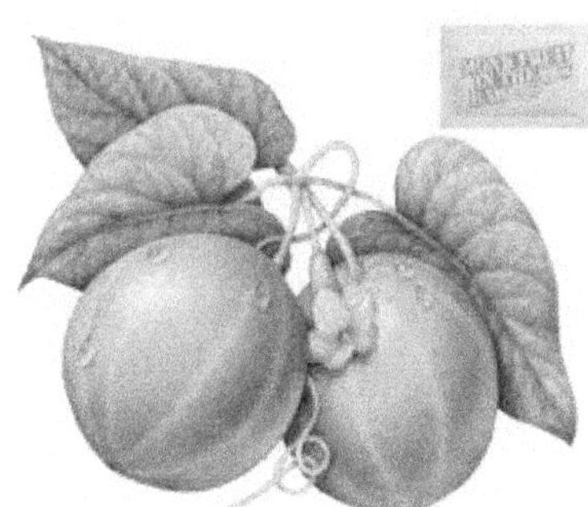

Lo Han is ready to use in the kitchen or on the coffee table. It is the main ingredient of a popular sweetener called In The Raw. Swanson Lo Han can be obtained via our web site, for around £13 a pot.

Diets That Work

Xylitol

This is a sugar alcohol occurring naturally in a variety of fruit and vegetables. Its used as a natural sugar-free sweetener and many nutritionists agree that it is a more natural and healthy alternative to sugar and other synthetic sweeteners.

Xylitol is ideal for anyone looking to an alternative to sugar in their diet and wanting to sweeten their food, beverages or supplements. Its also recommended by dentists as it helps reduce dental caries and tooth decay. You can buy Xylitol for around £20 for a 5 lb bag from many outlets – the web site has full details of easy ways to get it from reputable suppliers with free shipping.

Amazon stock one of the largest selections of sweeteners, both natural and artificial. You can see a good selection of most of them all collected together on one page by clicking a link on our website.

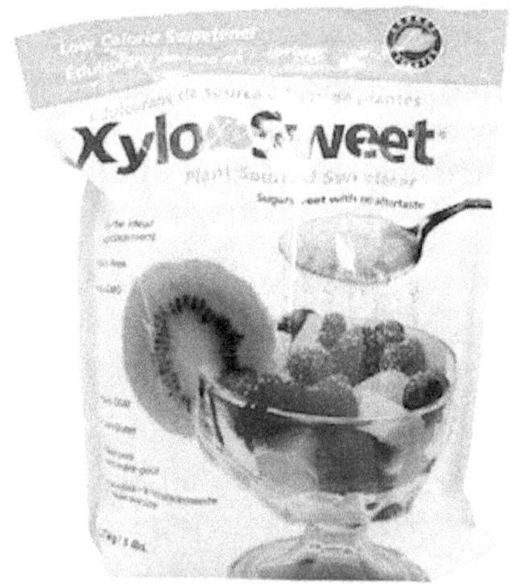

Are all the artificial sweeteners safe?

Artificial sweeteners are low-calorie or calorie-free chemical substances used instead of sugar to sweeten foods and drinks. They are found in thousands of products, from drinks, desserts and ready meals, to cakes, chewing gum and toothpaste. Find out what the NHS evidence says on the safety of some of the most common sweeteners approved for use in the UK

acesulfame K

aspartame

saccharin

sorbitol

sucralose

stevia (steviol glycosides)

xylitol

Cancer Research UK and the US National Cancer Institute have said that sweeteners don't cause cancer. "Large studies looking at people have now provided strong evidence that artificial sweeteners are safe for humans," says CR-UK.

All sweeteners available for use in the EU must first undergo a very rigorous safety assessment. These tests are conducted by the European Food Safety Authority (EFSA) before any food is allowed to be used in any food and drink for human consumption. As part of that trial and evaluation process, the EFSA sets a series of quantities called Acceptable Daily Intake (ADI). This is a maximum amount that tests have proved is safe to consume each day over the course of an average lifetime.

It's not necessary to keep track of how much of any particular sweetener products are being consumed each day, as everyone's eating habits are taken into consideration when specifying where the particular sweetener products can be used.

Diets That Work

Are sweeteners healthy?

Sweeteners may be pronounced safe, but the question you need to ask is "are they healthy?" Food manufacturers claim sweeteners help prevent tooth decay, control blood sugar levels and reduce our calorie intake. The EFSA has approved the health claims made about xylitol, sorbitol and sucralose, and many others, in relation to oral health and controlling blood sugar levels.

"Research into sweeteners shows they are perfectly safe to eat or drink on a daily basis as part of a healthy diet," says dietitian Emma Carder. She also says the products can be a useful alternative for people with diabetes who need to watch their blood sugar levels while still enjoying their favourite foods.

"Like sugar, most sweeteners provide a sweet taste but their biggest advantage and main difference is that, after consumption, they don't increase blood sugar levels," she says.

It has been suggested that the use of artificial sweeteners may have a stimulating effect on appetite and, therefore, may play a role in weight gain and obesity. Research into sweeteners however says otherwise. **There is little evidence from longer-term studies to show that sweeteners lead to increased energy intake or are likely to contribute to the risk of obesity.**

Artificial Sweeteners in soft drinks

Soft drinks are known by many names, sodas, pop, fizzy drinks and so on. Many proprietary names are also used such as Coke, which has become almost a generic term for cola flavoured drinks, though it's a registered name in every country in the world.

Those with a diabetes problem generally tend to use soft drinks made with artificial sweeteners as sugar upsets their blood glucose levels. Diabetes sufferers who need to avoid low blood sugar levels developing, as a result of their insulin medication, should be aware that most 'diet' flavoured soft drinks have a very low, or zero, sugar level and won't raise blood sugar levels. Always check the carbohydrate value on the drink if you are not sure particularly when trying a new brand of soft drink.

The Sweetener Book by Dr Eric Walters PhD

Which sweetener is really the best is a question asked by many calorie counting, health conscious shoppers. Like us you have probably been through a wide range of sweeteners and want to know what's best.

The 'best' sweetener depends on so many different factors: You may want a low glycemic index, one that doesn't upset your digestive system? Perhaps you have to consider high blood pressure?

This book looks at the scientific aspects of various sweeteners, their composition and any effects it has on our bodies and metabolism.

This book outlines all the pro's and con's of using sucrose, brown sugar, turbinado, molasses, fructose, glucose, lactose, high fructose corn syrup (HFCS), honey, agave nectar, sorbitol, lactitol, maltitol, mannitol, xylitol, fructo-oligosaccharides, inulin, tagatos, erythritol, glycerol, acesulfame, aspartame, and many more ingredients. How many of those are YOU familiar with?

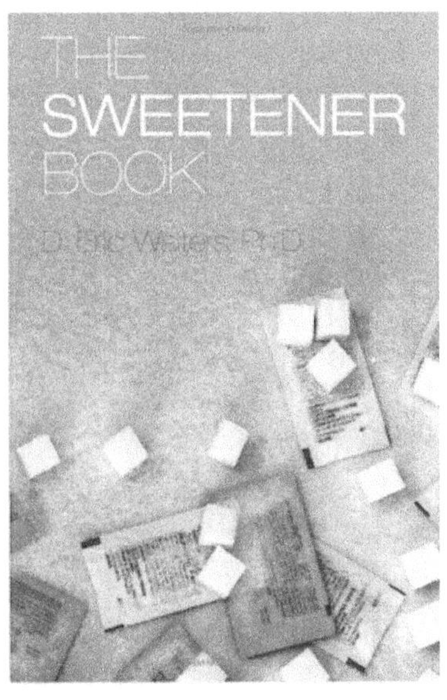

The Sweetener Book is an indispensible guide to the various types of sweetener being used in food today, its effects and value (or otherwise) to our health. You can obtain it via a link on the web site.

Diets That Work

Medical Studies

There have been many medical studies of the effects of artificial sweeteners in soft drink, but many of these studies are inconclusive. The results of such mixed findings. Diet soda may not be a healthy substitute for sugary soda.

For adults trying to wean themselves from sugary soda, diet soda is a possible short-term substitute, best used in small amounts over a short period of time. For children, the long-term effects of consuming artificially-sweetened beverages are unknown, so it's best for kids to avoid them.

There is a lot of conflicting research surrounding the health benefits of artificially sweetened drinks. Long-term studies show that regular consumption of artificially sweetened beverages reduces the intake of calories and promotes weight loss or maintenance, but other research shows no effect, and some studies even show weight gain.

A 2013 study showed that both sugar and artificially sweetened beverages were linked with an increased risk of developing Type 2 Diabetes.

One study of over 3,500 subjects looked at the long-term effects on weight. Participants were tracked for seven years and their body weights recorded. Those who drank artificially sweetened drinks had an almost fifty percent higher increase in BMI than those who did not use drinks with artificial sweeteners.

B   SUPPLEMENTS

Food supplements are concentrated sources of nutrients or other substances with a nutritional or physiological effect. They can be natural or man-made, and their purpose is to supplement the normal diet.

Supplements are usually added to make handling the food easier, or to increase the health benefits of the food. They can also be added to make the food easier to handle, to keep or to preserve it for longer, or to improve its appearance, such as with anti-oxidants. Some of the best known additives are Berberine, Creative, L-Cartine, Protein Powder, Fish Oil, and extracts of various plants.

Rosemary extract is increasingly added to products, such as beefburgers. This is not done to add flavour, as is traditionally done with fresh ground rosemary leaves on a joint of lamb for example. The rosemary extract has no taste, or colour and it is added as an anti-oxidant - to stop the meat from changing colour and going off. Everyone likes their beef burgers to look red, as this is perceived to be fresher or juicier.

Rosemary?

The herb Rosemary is found predominantly in the Alps, but has now spread all over the world. The usual folklore says that it takes its name from the Virgin Mary.

Legend says that she draped her cloak on a rosemary bush, and then placed a white flower on top of the cloak. The flower turned blue overnight, and the plant became known as the "Rose of Mary."

The Rosemary plant has been used for at least three thousand years and is found in cooking as a savory spice as well as now being used as a food preservative. It can also be used in the manufacture of cosmetics various beauty products. It is also becoming better known once again as a herbal medicine and is said to have positive effects on a wide range of health disorders.

Nature's Answer Rosemary Leaves

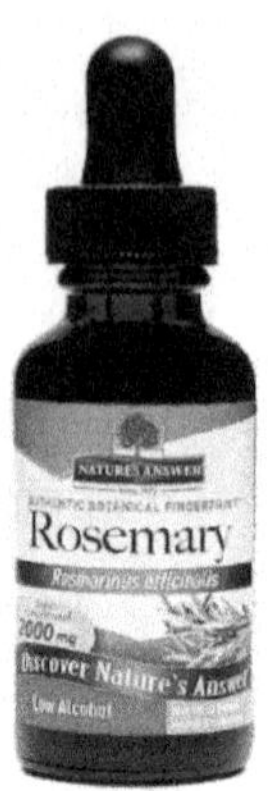

The organic alcohol extracts from *Nature's Answer* are produced using alcohol, water and coconut glycerin using their cold Bio-Chelated proprietary extraction process. This yields a holistically balanced and standardized extract.

Liquid extracts are absorbed into the body much faster than tablets or capsules and as such they are more potent than tinctures. You can order the **Nature's Larder Rosemary Leaves** via the web site.

Omega 3 Fish Oil

The 'Omega 3 fatty acids are very important to our bodies, and have all kinds of health benefits for the brain They help fight depression and anxiety) and joints such as knees.

High levels of blood fat can be reduced by fish oil supplements, thanks to the Omega 3 oily fish (such as smoked mackerel or haddock) is a great source of Omega 3 but many people don't get enough oily fish in their diet so adding the Omega 3 helps to counteract the deficiency.

One of the benefits of Omega 3 can be the reduction of non-alcoholic fatty Liver Disease (NAFLD) which is the most common cause of liver disease in the west. This and sixteen other ways that Omega 3 can help your body are explained on the Authority Nutrition page about the supplement.

Nu U Nutrition have Omega 3 Fish Oil 365 Softgel capsules available in handy bottles. These have maximum potency, come in high absorbency softgel capsules and NO fishy aftertaste. Manufactured in the UK to GMP standards, details can be found on the website in the Supplements section.

Many supplements contain active ingredients that can have strong effects in the body. Always be alert to all the side effects, especially when trying a new product. Always check the label and the small print on any accompanying leaflets.

The book about Supplements described below is a veritable mine of information about over 150 of the most commonly found supplements. With a copy of this book at hand you can be confident about all the additives and supplements you may discover and form your own decision before choosing to put them into your body.

Health Professional's Guide to Dietary Supplements

This reference helps dieters, students and health professionals find information about the scientific evidence for and against more than 120 popular dietary supplements. The supplements covered have been grouped into 12 chapters of the book based on their main desired effect, such as weight loss or enhancing sports performance.

Each supplement has been given one-to-five-star rating, based on the scientific evidence for the claimed effects. The guide discusses the crucial safety issues of each of the supplements covered. It also suggests recommended dosages for certain particular effects.

Each supplement covered has a short summary of its commonly stated effects and clinical evidence of any side-effects.

The ***Healthcare Professionals Guide to Supplements*** is an invaluable little reference book, available as a paperback from Amazon. The supplements that are covered in the guide are generally plant based but there are other supplements such as protein, vitamins and so on, included too.

Vitamins

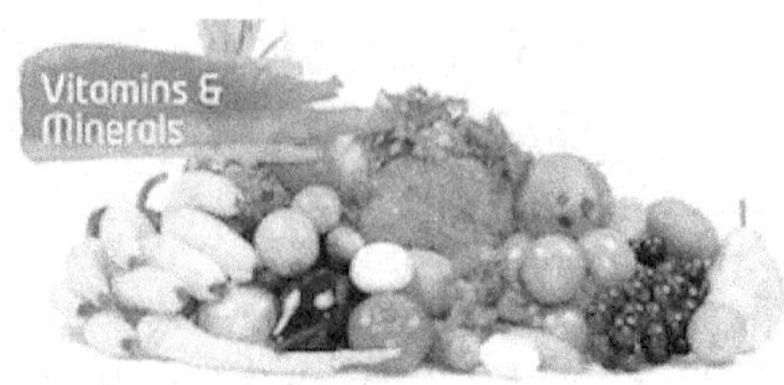

As well as the main food components of food, our bodies also need a wide variety of 'trace elements' to enable it to function. The main food ingredients are the following five types:

- Animal Products

- Fats and Oils

- Fruits

- Grains

- Seeds

The additional elements needed by our bodies to function properly and fight off germs and diseases are minerals such as nickel, copper, manganese and zinc, each of which have particular roles to play. Iron, for example, carries oxygen around the body in blood and is the main component responsible for the red colour in haemoglobin.

Trace elements are also essential nutrients that your body needs to work properly, but in much smaller amounts than vitamins and minerals. Trace elements are found in small amounts in a variety of foods such as meat, fish, cereals, milk and dairy foods, vegetables and nuts.

There are many occasions that the food we eat is deficient in certain vitamins and it can be beneficial to add vitamins to the food in the form of pills, powders or other ways in or on our food.

Diets that Work

Types of Vitamins

Vitamins can be conveniently split into two main groups, depending on which 'carrier' they are soluble in. There are water-soluble vitamins and fat-soluble vitamins.

Fat-soluble vitamins

Fat-soluble vitamins are found mainly in fatty foods and animal products, such as vegetable oils, milk and dairy foods, eggs, liver, oily fish and butter.

While your body needs these vitamins every day to work properly, you don't need to eat foods containing them every day.

This is because your body stores these vitamins in your liver and fatty tissues for future use. These stores can build up so they are there when you need them. However, if you have much more than you need, fat-soluble vitamins can be harmful.

Fat-soluble vitamins are: vitamins A, D, E and K.

Water-soluble vitamins

Water-soluble vitamins are not stored in the body, so you need to have them more frequently. If you have more than you need, your body gets rid of the extra vitamins when you urinate. As the body does not store water-soluble vitamins, these vitamins are generally not harmful.

Water-soluble vitamins are found in a wide range of foods, including fruit, vegetables, potatoes, grains, milk and dairy foods. Unlike fat-soluble vitamins, they can be destroyed by heat or being exposed to the air.

Some Water Soluble vitamins can also be lost in the water used for cooking. When we cook foods, especially if we boil them, we lose some of these vitamins. The best way to keep the water-soluble vitamins is to steam or grill foods, rather than boil them. Alternatively, use the cooking water in soups or in stews rather than pouring it away.

Fat-soluble vitamins are: Vitamin B, C and Folic acid.

Herbs

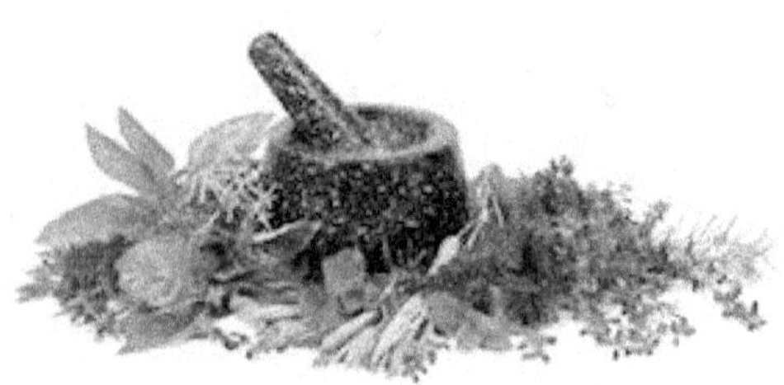

Herbs are any plants that are used for food, for flavouring, in medicine, or as fragrances (many herbs have savoury or aromatic properties).

In cooking herbs and spices are usually different things: HERBS usually means the leafy green or flowering parts of a plant (and they are encountered in cooking either fresh or dried), while SPICES are the product of other parts of the plant and are generally used as a dried product. Seeds are used as spices as are bark, roots and fruits, such as berries.

Herbs have a variety of uses including culinary, medicinal, and in some cases, spiritual. General usage of the term "herb" differs between culinary herbs and medicinal herbs. In medicinal or spiritual use any of the parts of the plant might be considered "herbs", including leaves, roots, flowers, seeds, root bark, inner bark (and cambium), resin and pericarp.

Their use to flavour food is well known, but many don't realise that they can also work as an anti-oxidant and that many have properties that will help in weight reduction. Too many would be dieters assume that any 'weight reduction' diet must consist solely of things like chicken or fish. They are missing out on some of the best and tastiest ingredients that can promote the loss of weight.

Among the best ways to improve the taste of food without adding any extra calories are herbs and spices. They also do

Diets that Work

so without adding sugars, or sodium, which can help ADD weight.

Many herbs and spices actually BOOST your metabolism, making your body burn off fat much more quickly. Among the hundreds of herbs and spices that can help you lose weight, these seem to work best. Here are a few of the best-known herbs that help in weight loss diets:

BLACK PEPPER

As well as the expected 'warming' properties, black pepper seeds have an ingredient that helps prevent the growth of new fat cells. It can be added to almost every food, but is especially good sprinkled in soups and even sweet foods such as yoghurt, oatmeal as well as over salads!

CARDOMAN

Cardoman is another thermo-genic spice often found in Indian cuisine. It tastes great when mixed with cinnamon, ginger or cloves in a curry or a chai tea. This citrusy spice can be added to confectionery, coffee and meats such as lamb.

CAYENNE

One of the most warming spices, Cayenne helps you boost your metabolism by increasing the body's heat and burn up calories. Just adding some cayenne to a meal can help you burn up to a hundred calories. Its excellent in soups, over eggs, for adding to dressings and dips for extra taste.

CINNAMON

This spice helps keep sugars in balance and is said to stop those cravings that often lead foodies to break away from their diet. Often encountered sprinkled on oatmeal, it can also be mixed into cottage cheese, yoghurt or hot drinks. Cinnamon also tastes great in rubs or marinades used on meats.

CUMIN

By adding cumin to food, this valuable herb could help triple the amount of fat you burn. Cumin can be found almost everywhere and can be used to add extra flavour to almost every type of food.

Diets That Work

DANDELION

Thought of by most people as simply a garden weed, it does have a lot of useful properties and has been drunk as an infusion (Dandelion Tea was once very popular). The roots as well as the leaves are used in cooking, even the bright yellow flowers are much cherished and can be used. Dandelion is now becoming common once again in kitchens as it is rich in several vitamins, including A, C and E and very high in minerals such as iron and potassium.

GARLIC

Although garlic can cause problems by lingering on the breath, it has been proven that consumption of even small traces of it in food will help your body burn off fat. It makes food much tastier, especially if its used raw - though this applies with all herbs and spices.

GINGER

Ginger is another spice that helps regulate blood sugars. It's ideal to help knock out those blips or spikes you find in glucose levels after you have eaten a meal rich in sugar or carbs. It has the same body warming (thermo-genic) qualities that cayenne and turmeric have. Try adding grated ginger into meals such as stir-fries, oven-baked fish or into tea. You will discover interesting new tastes and it should do you a lot of good too!

TURMERIC

A bright yellow spice that has been around for thousands of years, turmeric is a warming spice that actually increases body heat and so increases your metabolism. It is also thought to be helpful at many other things, such as fighting Alzheimer's disease. You can add it to heated foods such as soups, stews, roasted vegetables or nuts.

Diets that Work

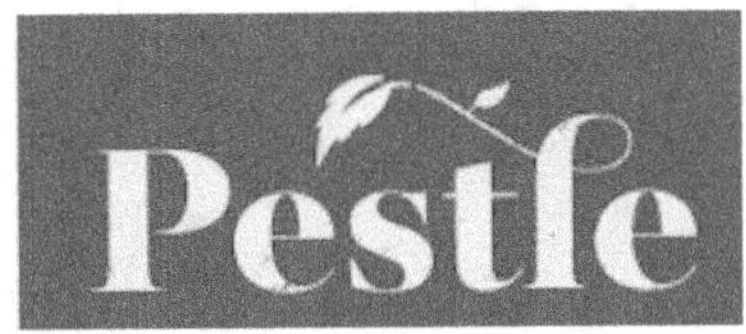

PESTLES are a UK company taking their inspiration from the natural origin of all medicines, perfumes and ingredients such as herbs. Pestle know exactly how certain herbs, correctly cultivated, can help with minor ailments, increase energy levels or help you to relax. Some herbs can even help to wash your clothes!

Pestles have one of the best selections of herbal products and will even teach you to grow some of the herbs yourself! Pestle Herbs have an e-commerce site for anyone who has lost faith in mainstream manufacturers of products for the body or the home.

The big companies so often offer products that have ingredients which are chosen for cost and not well-being. The products sold by Pestle are all essentially plant-based and contain only herbal ingredients. Each of the Pestles products have open, complete and honest ingredient information. In some cases these are based on easy to recreate recipes so that you can make their own versions.

Pestles dried herbs are all ethically-sourced, organic dried herbs and are hand-selected from the leading natural health and beauty brands such as *Urtekram, Bio Health, Potter's Herbals, Pukka* and *Weleda.*

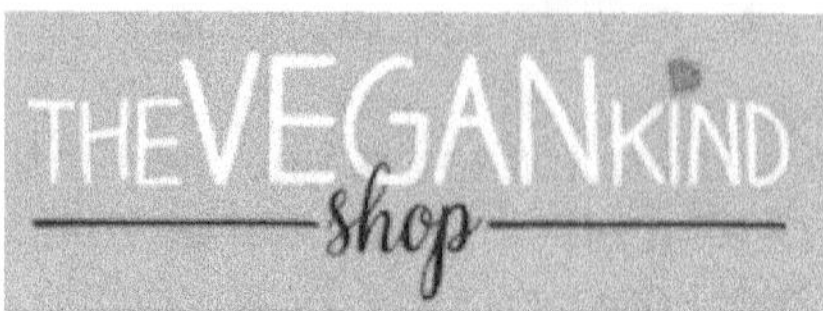

Another great source of herbal ingredients is a company in Glasgow called THE VEGAN KIND. Karris McCulloch is one of the co-founders and the Managing Director of TGF.

Karris has been a lifelong animal lover and passionate vegan. She wants to introduce as many people as possible of the huge benefits that Vegan life can bring and is making some amazing offers of introductory boxes of Vegan foods and Vegan beauty products.

 The Vegan Kind stock a full range of Vegan products and books, though many of the top Vegan titles are temporarily out of print, such is the demand. They also distribute a dozen much sought after supplements and vitamins, including *Omega 3, Spirulina, B12, Bilberry, Lecithin* and *Supergreens*.

Safflower

One herbal product not so well known is the Safflower. Of ten used in any weight loss diet is Safflower Oil, a natural, 100% pure energy-boosting extract that will promote a huge improvement in your body.

CLA Safflower Oil is a powerful extract that has been used for many years by professional athletes. It has grown a reputation for supporting lean muscle growth and fat removal, in both men and women.

A lot of the Safflower Oil supplements being sold only have a mere 10% CLA Safflower Oil; this is not really enough to start any real change. The CLA Safflower Oil being offered here contains 100% PURE CLA Safflower Oil. It can give you the results you are looking for to help you lose weight.

What is CLA Safflower Oil?

CLA Safflower Oil, is a powerful compound made from Safflowers. It's a polyunsaturated omega-6 fatty acid and is a colorless liquid at room temperature. Safflower Oil is the richest source of CLA (Conjugated Linoleic Acid) in the world.

Scientists and medical researchers have discovered that CLA Safflower Oil helps break down stored fat and increases lean muscle mass. This is one of the most incredible 'weight management' breakthroughs. Today it is helping men and women all over the world lose their belly fat and retain toned muscle naturally.

Now YOU can obtain this miraculous natural compound and achieve real weight loss. There is an offer of a **FREE** trial of 100% pure CLA Safflower Oil on our web site on the Safflower page.

Diets That Work

This is a premium quality CLA Safflower Oil which firstly promotes the breakdown of stored fat in the body, and secondly it encourages the body to keep the weight down.

CLA Safflower Oil also has been proved to promote the growth of lean muscle. The result is a healthy, highly toned body. CLA Safflower Oil is a great option for those looking for a product that uses only the best quality safflower oil and that helps achieve the very best results.

Linoleic Acid

The word Linoleic comes from the Greek word for flax, Linon with the oliec part, which means "obtained from olive oil". Linoleic acid is one of the two essential fatty acids, which the human body cannot synthesize from other food components. Linoleic Acid also has industrial uses and it is becoming widely used in beauty products thanks to its benefits to the skin: it is anti-inflammatory, reduces acne and helps retain moisture.

Conjugated Linoleic Acid ?

This is the main ingredient which is often thought of as the magic component in Safflower Oil. The CLAs are a group of several dozen isomers of Linoleic Acid (see below) that are found mostly in meat and dairy products.

The CLA Safflower Oil is made from vegetable oils, such as safflower. It is sold as a weight reducing and anti-cancer supplement. It is unsaturated.

There is medical evidence to support the claims that there is a beneficial effect in the use of Safflower Oil in weight reduction plans by moderately overweight dieters. Tests on farm livestock showed CLA promoted growth and prevented muscle wasting, with any fat produced being suppressed, due to a boost in energy expenditure.

(*Source: The Health Professional's Guide to Dietary Supplements by Shawn M. Talbot, and Kerry Hughes.*)

Diets that Work

Diet Drops

Diet Drops have long been a huge success in the USA; they have overtaken diet pills in the USA as the best selling slimming supplements. However, almost all of the American diet drops producers are unable to sell to the UK due to EU legislation on some of the ingredients.

Activ8 X are a British company who developed Diet Drops with a new formula, specially for the UK market. It is approved by the MHRA and is fully UK legal. Activ8 X was launched over 5 years ago and had hundreds of thousands of happy customers.

There have been many improvements directly resulting from the feedback that the UK distributors have received. Weight loss technology is always developing and improving and *HCG Slimming* now offer Diet Drops and similar products that have the best weight loss results on the market.

They offer a FREE 40 page guide containing recipes and tips to all their customers; details and links on the web site. The two parts of Gravit8 (Supersculpt & DietVits) work together in harmony to make losing weight a truly rewarding & enjoyable experience.

When using Gravitate, you no longer feel hungry, which is a huge bonus and helps tremendously in getting rid of your excess weight more easily. They really do work to suppress your hunger and those awful pangs you get when on a diet.

Diets That Work

Gravitate Nutrition

Compared to Activ8 X, Gravitate Nutrition is much easier to take, being in tablet form. There is no need to worry about counting drops. The kit contains two products to give you more weight loss power. Gravitate Nutrition also has a more powerful formula to provide stronger clinically proven appetite suppression. It is very straight forward to use and has a FREE easy to follow diet plan. The packages are good value and start at just £19.99.

Activ8 X has been a much-loved product for several years and has now been developed even further and replaced by Gravitate Nutrition. The distributors are so confident you'll love *Gravitate Nutrition* that all orders come with a 35-day money back guarantee!

Beware of counterfeit and fake Activ8 X bottles that were available for a time and could often be seen in some markets. The only genuine source is via mail order from the manufacturers – details on our web site. The official Activ8 X product has now been replaced with Gravitate Nutrition).

These have been specially formulated for men and women, and contain no caffeine or other stimulants. And no sugar of course. Their natural ingredients give no known side effects. They certainly make losing weight much easier. The Gravitate shake mixes complement the main Supersculpt and Divetvits products and are a really tasty, mouth-0watering, low calorie alternative to grazing on snacks.

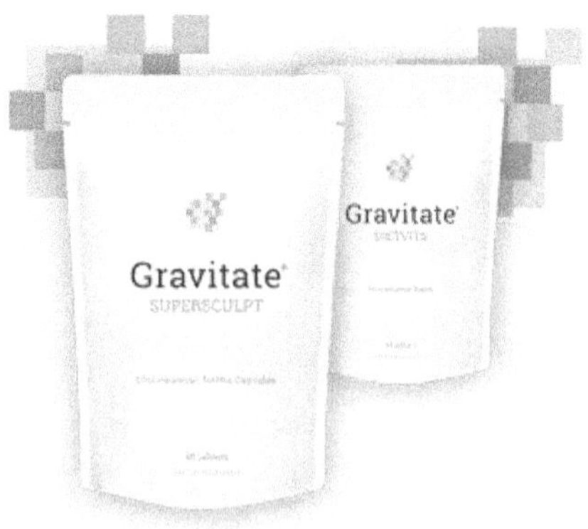

Slim Diet Patches

Diet patches are a great way of absorbing the widely renowned and highly regarded slimming properties of **fucus, acai berry** and **green tea** directly into your body. They work quicker and more efficiently as they do not have to pass through your digestive system, like tablets, pills or capsules. It's a great alternative to taking supplements orally.

The Slim Diet Patch from Bauer is a great new supplement that works differently to other supplements. You don't need to ingest it orally; that way a lot of the useful ingredients are lost in the digestive system. With tablets, pills and capsules your body only gets the benefit of a small fraction of the ingredients.

With the Slim Diet Patch's technology almost all the powerful fat-fighting ingredients are absorbed into your body, meaning you get the full benefit of the weight reducing ingredients.

With Slim Diet Patch, the active ingredients are in direct contact with your skin, allowing trans-dermal technology to deliver them straight into your body instead of going through your digestive system. Unlike pills or capsules, the effects of which don't last long, the Slim Diet Patch releases a steady stream of its powerful ingredients over a period of 24 hours, helping you lose weight day and night, wherever you are and whatever you're doing.

All you need do is attach one Slim Diet Patch on your skin, just like a sticking plaster, in the morning and you can then forget all about it. The weight reducing ingredients in a patch are absorbed by the body over the following 24 hours. This gives you 'round the clock' weight loss, all day and all night. Bauer offer a 100% secure order line with a two-month guarantee.

Diets That Work

Slim Diet Patches contain three main ingredients:

Fucus (Seaweed Extract)

A key ingredient in many homeopathic medicines the extract is taken from kelp found in seas and river estuaries. Fucus is rich in vitamins, in antioxidants and minerals.

The Fucus in the Slim Diet Patches is iodine-rich which helps make certain that you have enough energy to get through the day and any exercise. Iodine stimulates the thyroid, the part of the body that controls our metabolism. When the thyroid is stimulated by the Fucus, it boosts your metabolic rate and helps to burn a lot of the stubborn fat stored around the body. If you are deficient in iodine it makes you feel tired and lethargic.

Euterpe Oleracea (Acai Fruit Extract)

Acai is another natural ingredient that helps you lose weight. Inside Acai are essential fatty acids, amino acids and phytosterols which all burn fat more efficiently, leading to quicker weight loss.

The essential fatty acids Omega-3 and Omega-6 in Acai also boost the metabolism, which of course burns fat much more efficiently. Amino acids are very useful in helping the body to recover after exercise. Phytosterols help the body improve its efficiency and better absorb nutrients.

Camellia Sinensis (Green Tea Leaf Extract)

Green tea contains lots of natural ingredients that benefit your body's health and helps with weight loss. Ingredients in green tea include antioxidants, such as catechins, which protect cells.

One of these catechins, EGCG, has been proven to help the body's cells to break down fat. Another way it helps with the metabolism is by thermogenesis. This is the increase in the body's temperature which helps burn off the fat.

Diets that Work

Phen 375

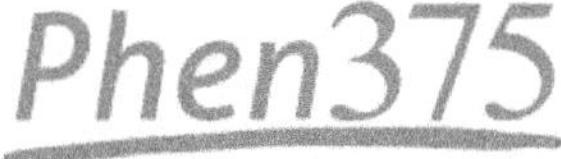

Phen375 is made from ingredients selected to help weight loss, by suppressing cravings and hunger. Eating lots of extra calories will add to your weight unless burned off. Phen375 can also provide specifically-devised diet plans and exercise routines.

All the weight loss experts, be they doctors, dieticians or other experts, are all agreed that the best way to lose weight is to eat fewer calories and generally be more active. For most people, a reasonable goal is to lose about a pound a week.

For most people, to do that you need to take in about 500 calories a day less than you do now. Quite easily done by simply eating a range of nutritious foods and doing some regular exercise! Phen375 can help you achieve this.

What's in Phen 375?

L-Carnatine tartrate dissolves your stored body fat.

Anhydrous caffeine reduces hunger, and cravings.

Coleus Forskolii Root PE (10% Forskolin): Activates adenylyl cyclase and raises cyclic AMP levels in cells.

Citrus Aurantium: increases the body's metabolism.

Cayenne Pepper: has thermogenic powers which increase your temperature and helps to burn up more calories

Dendrobium Nobile Extract This is an antipyretic plant alkaloid which is made from orchids and improves digestion.

C   DIETS

There are hundreds if not thousands of different diets and it can be very confusing when faced with so many, especially some of the 'flash in the pan' 'faddish' ones that last for a very short time. We have no intention of describing them all, some don't warrant any inclusion at all, though the omission of any should not automatically be taken as a dismissal of them.

This **Diets That Work** book covers only those ones that we KNOW are "Diets that Work". Almost all these diets have been tried by us personally and can confirm that we have seen weight loss as a result. Here are some of the best weight reduction diets in summary – see the pages further on in the book for more details of each diet.

Warrior DIET

The Warrior Diet was created by Ori Hofmekler and it seems to work best with some periods of intensive exercise, but refraining from eating during the day, and then eating as much as is desired during a four hour period in the evening. The food choices are based on whole organic foods, plants and meat; you must strictly avoid processed and artificially manufactured food.

Paleo Diet

The Paleo diet is based on emulating the diet of our hunter-gatherer ancestors. It includes wholesome but unprocessed foods that resemble what they look like in nature. Our ancestors thrived eating basic and unprocessed foods and had no modern day diseases and problems, such as obesity, diabetes and heart disease.

Diets that Work

SIRT Diet

The SIRT diet is one of the latest diet crazes that so many people seem to be talking about. According to researchers, these special foods work by activating specific proteins in the body called sirtuins. There are many sirtuins, please check on our SIRT diet page for more information.

Low GL Diet

GL stands for Glycaemic Load. It's a unit of measurement that tells you exactly what a particular food will do to your blood sugar. Foods with the highest Glycaemic Load levels have a much greater effect on your blood sugar, which isn't at all wanted. It's important to know what those foods are. On the other hand, those foods with a low GL will more easily encourage the body to burn fat. That is the ideal situation in reducing weight.

Caveman Diet

This is very similar to the Warrior Diet mentioned above, and described more fully below.

Glycemic Diet (GI)

Cuts out foods that have a high GI index and so balances blood sugars and insulin, helping fat burn.

Diets That Work

Grapefruit Diet

Was called the 'Hollywood diet' for many years. Anyone taking any medication should beware that enzymes in grapefruit can have bad side effects.

Cabbage Soup Diet

Some people can't abide cabbage, others love it. You get to enjoy(endure?) a whole week of only cabbage soup on this diet, and can shed about ten pounds doing that.

3 Hour Diet

Limits eating food to every few hours, but allows red meat, chocolate, chicken and bacon! There are several derivatives of this and it bears a lot of resemblance to the **Celebrity Diets** that get huge publicity, under the names of many movie and music stars.

Skinny Bitch Diet

a no-nonsense, tough-love guide for savvy girls who want to stop eating crap and start looking fabulous. This is done by cutting out sugar, meat, dairy, flour, caffeine and alcohol.

Celebrity Diets

Many of today's film and music stars are associated with particular diets. Some of the best known are Beyonce, Halle Berry, Angelina Jolie and Jeniffer Lopez.

All these stars invariably have stunning bodies and are pretty universally admired and each has amazingly gorgeous bodies. Due to the demands on their time, they tend to eat small meal, but eat, or rather graze, frequently throughout the day. Instead of eating three big meals, they snack every 2-3 hours. This is the basis of almost all celebrity diets that work.

Diets that Work

According to the diet gurus, several small meals a day is an excellent way to boost the body's metabolism, which invariably will lead to weight loss. Taking on small amounts of food every three hours or so has led to this routine being called the Three Hour Diet.

It is the basis of almost every diet used by bodybuilders who are experts at losing fat. This method of dieting is of great assistance in curbing cravings for particular food cravings, especially the sugar rich food, and it makes sure that the dieter doesn't go hungry.

Hunger is the greatest enemy of the dieter. Not feeling those pangs of hunger enables them to stay on the diet and keep their cravings under control.

The Zone Diet

This is yet another diet that is very similar to the Three Hour Diet, in that it spreads out three meals throughout the day with additional snacks taken in between. The Zone Diet tries to achieve a balance between the body's hormones by use of a food plan with a strict percentage of nutrients: 30% protein, 30% fat and 40% carbs. No processed foods are allowed on this diet - burgers are barred as are all kinds of junk foods.

The High Protein Diet is also very similar to the Zone diet, as it follows the basic mantra of a balance of food types. It is most often said to be one of the Celebrity Diets That Work. Many athletes follow this diet, as do Jennifer Anniston and Demi Moore.

Diets That Work

Atkins Diet & South Beach Diet

In the well-known **Atkins Diet,** you control the amount of carbs you consume and only eat wholesome foods. As it's high in fat some physicians and nutritionists warn that the fat consumption required by these diets can be excessive, and potentially dangerous. Qualified medical advise should be obtained first before embarking on an Atkins Diet.

The **South Beach Diet** is a modified carbo-hydrate system, often called a modified Atkins Diet, but with three distinct phases. It's a low-carb diet which is similar to the Low GL Diet (discussed below). It tries to achieve a balance of 'good' and 'bad' cabs and has a difficult First Stage where many food types are banned, but then reintroduced later.

The South Beach Diet was developed by cardiologist Dr. Arthur Agatston in the mid 1990s and promoted heavily. He had noticed that Atkins was working for some of his patients but was reluctant to approve it for anyone with cardiac problems, so divided this originally as an eating plan which included fibre and lean protein.

South Beach was heavily promoted by Dr Agatston's book in 2002 and became known as a fad diet that has lots of Low GL and high fibre ingredients, as well as lean protein. The book that launched and promotes the South Beach Diet has several discredited claims and some faults. There have been concerns over its long term safety, but an entire industry has developed around food companies delivering meals to homes that follow the South Beach Diet. Many of the diet's guidelines are based on sensible principles you will find discussed elsewhere on our web site.

There is now a SUPERCHARGED version of the SouthBeach Diet that seems to have addressed most of the concerns about the launch book. The South Beach Diet certainly does fall into the categories of those *Diets That Work*.

Diets that Work

A new version of the original million-copy best seller and the Good Carbs Bad Carbs Guide. The new South Beach Diet Supercharged increases weight loss by adding a unique 3-phase exercise plan.

The principles of the diet in the Supercharged version are essentially the same - Phase 1 giving you a short, sharp weight loss if you need to lose more than 10 pounds. Phase 2 addresses a reduction in calorie intake and helps you achieve a good balance while Phase 3 is all about keeping up the diet and the weight loss, as diet maintenance.

The Supercharged South Beach Diet has had exercises added to it enabling you to burn more fat much more quickly. This is designed to achieve permanent weight loss and an improvement in your health. The new Supercharged book by Dr Agatston and his dietician colleague Joseph Signorie is available now as are his many other supporting books, such as the **South Beach Diet Cookbook** (I really recommend this one as it contains some wonderful tasty recipes).

Warrior Diet

What is it?

The Warrior Diet was created by Ori Hofmekler and it seems to work best with some periods of intensive exercise, but refraining from eating during the day, and then feast in the evening. Food choices are based on whole foods, plants and meat, but avoiding processed and manufactured food.

The basis of the Warrior Diet is to eat simply as an old time soldier from hundreds of years ago would have eaten. You fast by day but eat as much you wish after dark.

 In fact even the daytime period is not all fast as you are allowed to graze, mainly on fruit such as berries, nuts and vegetables. At night you are allowed as much vegetables, protein and carbs as you wish.

The Warrior Diet is quite unlike any other diet we have ever come cross. The idea is that it accelerates the metabolism and burns fat. In addition to burning up fat it also builds muscle strength.

The Warrior Diet, devised by Ori Hofmekler, doesn't demand that you count calories at all, nor are there specific strict food lists. You can skip the daytime grazing if you wish, or keep them to a minimum. What is suggested is alternating between 'minimum eating' phases during the day and then 'overeating phases' in the evening. According to the Warrior Diet's official web site this promotes the best hormonal environment, improves your energy production and fat burning.

The Warrior Diet asks you to follow your instinct when it comes to dieting. You should not be swayed by processed foods or the everyday and generally accepted rules as to what types of calories and macronutrients to eat and especially WHEN to eat them. Instead, you must learn to eat like an ancient warrior -- ancient warriors had very little at all to eat during the day and instead ate their "hunt" at night.

Diets that Work

The deviser of the Warrior Diet advocates controlled fasting and exercising on a virtually empty stomach. You ease into having your food intake consist primarily of only one meal a day. If you adapt to the diet in the way Ori Hofmekler claims you will, you'll be better able to burn fat for fuel, have greater energy and you'll become lean without counting calories.

The Warrior Diet book (details below) written by the system's deviser, Mr Ori Hofmekler, advocates exercise as part of the plan, recommending total body strength training with moves such as press-ups, squats and high jumps. You are encouraged to include short bursts of high-intensity cardio activity, such as sprints and frog jumps, in these intense sessions that last only 20 to 45 minutes.

Original Warrior Diet book *by Ori Hofleker*
The Warrior Diet is proving increasingly popular and is much talked about. Nomads, hunters, the Greeks, and the Romans all based their consumption on survival science and Ori Hofleker's book suggests a rather radical but very simple lifestyle.

Combining historical information and scientific studies the author points out that robust health and a lean, strong body is most easily got by assuming the classical warrior lifestyle of working and eating sparingly during the day and then feasting after dark.

Specific elements from the Warrior Diet Nutritional Programme reshape not just the body but also your mind and the brain's expectations. The book's chapters cover typical warrior meals and recipes; sex drive and potency. Sections of the diet are also aimed at women. It shows you how to attain enduring vigor, explosive strength, a better appearance and increased vitality and health.

The current edition of the Warrior Diet book is 420 pages long and can be hard to find. We can point you to stocks and Ori Hofmekler's other best selling book, *Maximum Muscle, Minimum Fat.* It's all about the secret science of physical transformation and is reading for anyone serious about muscle tissue.

Diets That Work

JAMIE EASON

Often called the 'smartest woman alive" and certainly one of the fittest, Jamie Eason follows the Warrior Diet. Jamie is a model, a fitness trainer and a figure Pro, and has her own fitness system and has a store selling her 'Signature Series' of plans, accessories, work-out equipment and multi-vitamin pills.

Jamie is a cancer survivor, model, fitness enthusiast, mother, and wife. Her *LiveFit* trainer, articles and recipes have helped thousands of people get fit and change their lives.

She's proven time and time again that weights and building muscle are not only for men. Women all over the world have followed Jamie's lead. Jamie continues to write articles, model, and star in video trainers.

Paleo Diets

Eating the Natural Way

The Paleo Diet is based on emulating the diet of our hunter-gatherer ancestors. It includes unprocessed foods that resemble what they look like in nature. Our ancestors thrived eating basic and unprocessed foods. They were generally free of many modern day diseases and problems, such as obesity, diabetes and heart disease. The paleolithic age humans ate whatever foodstuffs that mother nature was making available at the time. Some ate a low-carb diet while others ate a high-carb diet with lots of plants. Listed below are the main Paleo Diet 'food rules'

A. EAT

Grass-fed, pasture raised and organic foods are the best foods for you, if they are affordable. If not, then just make sure to always go for the least processed option. 'Fair Game' are all real, unprocessed Paleo foods, such as meats, fish, eggs, veg, fruits, nuts, seeds, herbs, spices, healthy fats and oils.

Meats: Beef, lamb, chicken, turkey, pork etc.

Fish and Seafood: Salmon, trout, haddock, shrimp, shellfish, etc. Choose wild-caught if you can.

Eggs: Choose free-range, pastured or omega-3 enriched eggs.

Vegetables: Broccoli, kale, peppers, onions, carrots, tomatoes, etc.

Fruits: Apples, bananas, oranges, pears, avocados, strawberries, blueberries and more.

Tubers: Potatoes, sweet potatoes, yams, turnips, etc.

Nuts and Seeds: Almonds, macadamia nuts, walnuts, hazelnuts, sunflower seeds, pumpkin seeds and more.

Healthy Fats and Oils: Lard, tallow, coconut oil, olive oil, avocado oil and others.

Diets That Work

Salt and Spices: sea salt, garlic, turmeric, rosemary, etc.

B AVOID

All processed foods, sugar, soft drinks, artificial sweeteners, most dairy products, legumes, grains, vegetable oils, margarine and trans fats. You should especially avoid all these ingredients, found in many modern dishes, especially in restaurants.

Sugar and Corn Syrup (Soft drinks, fruit juices, table sugar, candy, pastries, ice cream and many others).

Grains: Includes breads and pastas, wheat, spelt, rye, barley, etc.

Legumes: beans, lentils etc

Dairy: Avoid most dairy, especially low-fat (some versions of Paleo dishes do have full-fat dairy like butter and cheese).

Vegetable Oils: Soybean oil, sunflower oil, cottonseed oil, corn oil, grape seed oil, safflower oil and others.

Trans Fats: Found in margarine and various processed foods. Usually referred to as "hydrogenated" or "partially hydrogenated" oils.

Artificial Sweeteners: Aspartame, Sucralose, Cyclamates, Saccharin, Acesulfame Potassium. Wherever possible you should try to use natural sweeteners instead, such as *LoHan* (Monk Fruit), honey or Xylitol which is made from plant alcohol. .

Highly Processed Foods: (Everything labeled "diet" or "low-fat" or has many weird ingredients).

C. DRINKS ALLOWED ON A PALEO DIET

Glass of water

> When it comes to hydration, pure water is essential for your metabolism and should always be your drink of choice.

> The following drinks aren't exactly Paleo, but most people drink them and you should note the following

> **Tea** is very healthy and loaded with antioxidants and various beneficial compounds. Green tea is best.

> **Coffee** is actually very high in antioxidants as well. Studies show that it has many health benefits. Irregular coffee can have less caffeine than regular so is unlikely to have much effect on heart rate, but it should only be drunk in moderation.

Sensible Indulgences when on a Paleo Diet

The following items are often regarded as bad, however they are also a part of many diets, and are perfectly healthy, when consumed in small reasonable amounts:

> **Wine:** Quality red wine is high in antioxidants and beneficial nutrients.

> **Dark Chocolate:** Choose one that has 70% or higher cocoa content. Quality dark chocolate is very nutritious and extremely healthy.

Diets That Work

Paleo Cookbooks

These amazing books show you how to cook the most delicious and nutritious meals from the tastiest & healthiest ingredients

The paleo diet is not one that has been devised or designed by diet doctors, faddishists, or nutritionists; it is a diet designed by nature!

Paleo diets is not the latest weight loss program or celebrity diet that leaves you craving sugar-laden foods. Remember, they are in fact the same food that our ancestors ate!

Paleo Cookbooks is a total collection of hundreds of Nikki Young's favourite Paleo-friendly recipes. They have been chosen to help you follow the healthiest and most nutritious diet in the world.   These cookbooks contain **NONE** of the following:

- Grains
- Potatoes
- Lentils
- Dairy
- Processed Sugars
- Preservatives

Paleo recipes result in healthy meals that do not result in you eating bland, boring or tasteless foods. You cook with fresh ingredients that provide the ultimate range of delicious flavors that will have anyone rushing to the kitchen to eat your next meal. The Paleo meal recipes in the cookbooks also include desserts that aren't overloaded with sugar and white flour, which are the very ingredients that all too often leave you bloated, or feeling fatigued after eating.

With the **Paleo Books Package** you can enjoy eating 375 simple and easy to create Paleo recipes including 8 recipe categories and 5 special recipe categories not limited to chocolate and Paleo breakfast recipes!

Diets that Work

You will be able to create Paleo recipes that help you to stay away from unhealthy sweets and fried foods! You will receive the three bonus guides:

Paleo Guide To Getting Started,

Paleo Eating Out Guide

Paleo Food Guide

These three books will help you understand the Paleo diet and keep you on the path to following a healthier diet and enjoying improved health. You will also receive the 30-day Paleo Meal Plan that you can follow to fast-track your health, energy, vitality, weight loss and achieve many other health benefits associated with following the Paleo diet.

The package also includes the Four Ingredients Paleo Cookbook. In this Cookbook there are 65 delicious Paleo recipes, all using only FOUR ingredients. It's yours absolutely free – you can find full details of it on the Paleo page on the web site.

1000 RECIPE BOOK PACKAGE

There are 1000 Paleo Recipes in another package of books from Matt and the team at Paleo Valley. The books cover all kinds of cooking and there are separate volumes on Fish, Chicken, Pork, stews and a great book about Paleo Desserts. This is the largest collection of Paleo recipes we have seen; each of the recipes are dense in nutrients. This could save you thousands each year on hiring your own Paleo chef – you CAN do this yourself.

Diets That Work

The Paleo Primer

The **PALEO PRIMER** is a jump-start guide to losing body fat and living primally. The authors, have assembled advice and tips on how you can re-shape your life, your eating and your body. Its done by eating as our ancestors did.

If you want to try living primally but are not sure where to begin, this is a great book to launch your Paleo diet as simply and quickly as possible. It offers clear guidance, easily understood explanations and some very tasty recipes. Its written by renowned fitness experts Keris Marsden and Matt Whitmore who can help you transform your body just by making changes to your food.

The Paleo Primer shows you how to:

- Lose fat without losing muscle

- Get clear, glowing skin

- Balance your moods

- Boost concentration

- Feel fit and full of energy

-

There are over 100 paleo recipes in this book, plus shopping lists and nutrition tips; a great guide to a healthy and enjoyable lifestyle. Full information is on the web site.

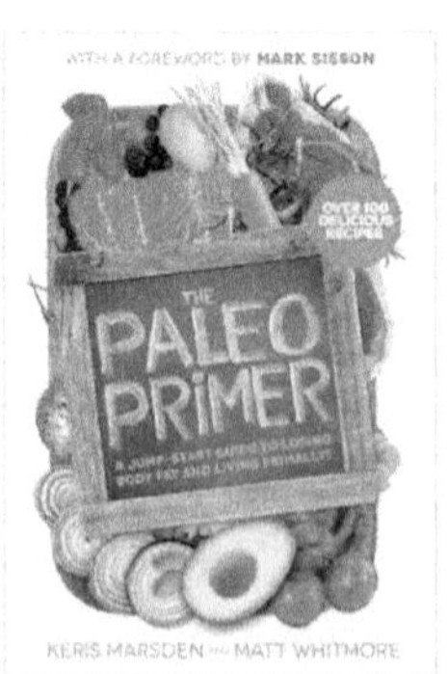

SIRT Diet

The SIRT diet is one of the latest diet crazes that so many people seem to be talking about.   According to researchers, these special foods work by activating specific proteins in the body called sirtuins. The most common of the SIRT FOODS are:

- Green Tea
- Dark Chocolate
- Parsley
- Capers
- Red Wine
- Kale
- Turmeric
- Citrus
- Fruits
- Apples
- Blueberries

SIRTUINS

Sirtuins are thought to protect cells in the body and prevent them from dying which often happens when cells are under stress. It's thought that sirtuins regulate inflammation, the metabolism as well as the aging process.

It's also believed that sirtuins influence the body's ability to burn fat and that they may do this by boosting the body's metabolism. This can lead to a drop of as much as seven pounds in weight in ONE WEEK, while continuing to maintain muscle strength.

Diets That Work

Composition of a Sirt Diet

Aidan Goggins and Glen Matten's SIRT diet has two distinct phases:

PHASE 1 lasts for only one week. Calories are restricted to 1000kcal for three days. This is done by drinking three SIRTfood green juices and one meal each day. Both are rich in SIRTfoods. The juices usually include kale, celery, rocket, parsley, green tea and lemon.

Typical meals are turkey escalope with sage, capers and parsley, chicken and kale curry and prawn stir fry with noodles.

From days four to seven, the intake is increased to 1500kcal, invariably comprising two SIRTfood green juices and two meals rich in SIRTfood each day.

PHASE 2 is the maintenance phase and it last for 14 days. In Phase 2 the weight continues to reduce, but steadily.

The SIRT Diet's designers claim it is a sustainable and realistic way to reduce weight. They say that weight loss is not the prime focus of the diet and that it has been designed to use the best foods nature has to offer.

They recommend a longer term diet which involved eating THREE balanced SIRTfood rich meals every day with one of the prescribed SIRT food green juices.

SIRT Food Diet Book

The revolutionary plan for health and weight loss
by Aiden Goggins & Glen Matten

The official Sirt Food Diet is a pretty revolutionary way to lose seven pounds in just 7 days. This book will help you substitute your regular food and drink with healthy SIRT food. It promises effective and sustained weight loss plus a huge increase in energy and glowing health!

Switch on your body's hidden powers to burn away fat, and boost your weight loss; It's claimed that you can stave off disease with the SIRT DIET which is easy-to-follow and has been developed by Aiden Goggins and Glen Matten who are experts in nutritional medicine.

Dark chocolate, coffee, kale - these are all foods that activate sirtuins and switch on the so-called 'skinny gene' pathways in the body. The same pathways more commonly activated by fasting and exercise, they help the body to burn fat, increase overall muscle strength and improve your all-round health.

In their initial trials an increase in lean muscle was noticed as well as consistent weight loss averaging seven pounds over the course of just a week! This is the only book stemming from their research, which was carried out to strict scientific standards.

Low GL Diet

GL stands for Glycaemic Load. It's a unit of measurement that tells you exactly what a particular food will do to your blood sugar. Foods with the highest Glycaemic Load levels have a much greater effect on your blood sugar, which isn't at all wanted. It's important to know what those foods are.

On the other hand, those foods with a low GL will more easily encourage the body to burn fat. That is the ideal situation in reducing weight.

 Keeping the levels of blood sugar and the balance between them is the key concept at the core of the low GL Diet. Once that is achieved then sustainable weight loss will follow.

The GL Diet has often been described as "the perfect way to lose weight, gain energy and improve your overall health." Patrick Holford's revolutionary **Low GL Diet** is based on achieving a good balance of your blood sugars and is one of the safest and most effective ways to lose weight.

This is a truly effective, easy-to-follow diet that will not only help you lose weight and put an end to cravings, but also seems to noticeably boost your energy and improve your health, just as Patrick Holford said it will.

THE LOW-GL DIET MADE EASY

This handy book explains the revolutionary Glyceamic Load (GL) system and tells you which foods are low-GL 'heroes' and which foods you should avoid, how to get started, portion size and how to add up your GL count. The book also has a very comprehensive three-week action plan. It includes shopping lists, day-by-day menus and some delicious mouth-watering recipes.

THE LOW-GL DIET MADE EASY book is a great read and a good manual if you are looking for a way to lose weight safely and effortlessly.

Patrick Holford, BSc, DipLON, FBANT, NTCRP, is a pioneer in several radical new approaches to food, health and nutrition.

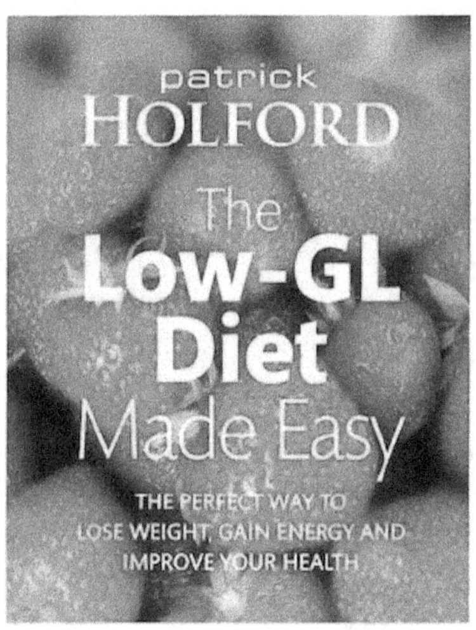

The Low GL DIET COOKBOOK
Food GLorious Food !

by Patrick Molford

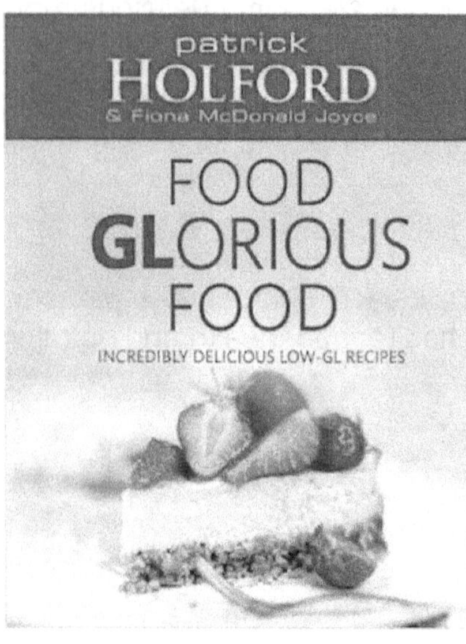

In the strictest sense of the word, Food **GL**orious Food is neither a diet nor a cookbook. It sets out to be a celebration of the many and various ingredients that can everyone enjoy a much healthier diet.

This is no tough dietary regime though - the recipes are delicious and exciting and have the added advantage of being low GL too. That means you - and your guests - can enjoy meals that are both deeply satisfying and health enriching.

Written in association with Fiona McDonald Joyce, who specialises in healthy food that doesn't compromise on taste, **Food GLorious Food** is filled with dishes that will impress family and friends - without the need to resort to creamy sauces, sugar-laden concoctions or overly complex cooking techniques. With everything from curries to healthy roasts and gluten-free chocolate brownies, good food is firmly on the menu.

This book is essential reading for anyone who wants to feel and look healthier and boost energy levels, without disappointing their taste buds. If you want to keep eating great tasty food and diet at the same time, the book **Food GLorious Food** can be found on our web pages with others about the GL Diet.

Diet Systems

There are even more regimes and systems of diets than there are types of diet, some are terrific, some are just so-so, and some appear to have little or no effect. It can be a nightmare assessing which ones are worth the time spent trying them. We hope to relieve you of the burden and point you towards some that ARE worthwhile.

We enrolled various diets over a period on and interviewed others who had tried various 'led' courses where a qualified trainer is both in charge of the conduct of the course and provides ongoing advice.

This type of 'led' course is probably the best, especially if you have previously not had much success on diets, as that extra help can help keep you on track as well as provide ongoing mentoring and support.

- Danette May
- Hairy Bikers
- Bodyweight Burn
- Carbs After Dark

Other diet evaluations are still ongoing, and we shall publish the results as soon as these are available.

Danette May

Danette is America's leading fitness guru, who can help YOU love the body you live in. She is a certified personal trainer and a qualified nutritionist who has a safe and effective method to burn belly fat and look 10 pounds leaner in just 10 days!

Over the last 15 years she has helped hundreds of thousands of people around the world get into shape. Danette's web site has hundreds of free recipes to help you achieve your goal. She is also a mom with 3 kids!

7 Day Jumpstart

Lose 7 pounds in 7 days – SERIOUSLY! What's more, you will keep it off too! With this easy to follow step-by-step system you can jump-start your sluggish metabolism and melt away the fat. You will reduce the inflammation inside your body, increase your physical performance (no matter what age you are), revive and enhance your sex life, unlock unlimited energy and end your food cravings in minutes.

Danette's seven day programme will give you outrageous results without any paid and all achievable in the shortest time possible. Follow it exactly and you will instantly melt fat, boost your metabolism and look and feel more youthful and energetic.

No impossible exercises   **No** crazy food diets

No counting calories or carbs   **No** starvation

Burning Belly Fat.

 When it comes to eating for weight loss, there are 2 simple rules you MUST follow and they are probably not what you think!

Never skip a meal - breakfast, lunch or dinner

Never forget the snacks between meals.

Diets that Work

Three Day Detox

Have you got 3 days?

That's all it takes. Just 3 days !

Three days to get rid of the dangerous toxins and flush poisonous substances out of your body! Boost your energy levels fast so you don't feel wiped out and utterly exhausted all the time.

Harmful toxins get into your body through the pesticides that are found on your food, in your water, and as a part of many soaps and shampoos, cosmetics, fragrances. Even the air and fumes in our cities that you breathe in all the time.

The sad fact is, that you can't just get away from toxins; — toxins are EVERYWHERE. Undo the damage that toxins do. Transform your body with a detox.

The **Bikini Body Detox** is a natural, nutritious and cleansing programme. This will give your body exactly what you need top flush out all the toxins and boost your metabolism at the same time. It's unlikely that you've ever used anything like this before. It's a proven 7 day program to give you outrageous results in the shortest time possible. Follow it exactly and you will instantly melt fat, boost your metabolism and look and feel more youthful and energetic.

The **Bikini Body Detox** is not like so many other programs, which leave you grumpy and hungry or require you to resort to powdery shakes, pills and expensive equipment.

Danette May's
Bikini Body Recipes

To lose weight, you must eat properly. It sounds simple, but the truth is, if it were easy, many of us wouldn't be overweight.

The problem is that if you eat the wrong food, bad things can happen. You won't get the results. You'll waste your time. You'll feel discouraged and like many others before you, you will easily give up.

If you don't eat enough food, bad things can also happen: as well as sabotaging your health and dieting, you will probably encounter uncontrollable cravings and hunger pangs. You're likely to succumb to the feeling that it's all just a little bit too hard and will probably give up.

This is where Bikini Body Recipes comes in: It's a revolutionary fat loss strategy that has been proven to work. It does this by giving you a variety of delicious-tasting fat-burning recipes that not only taste great but they are easy and quick to make — in fact they take only 10 minutes to prepare!

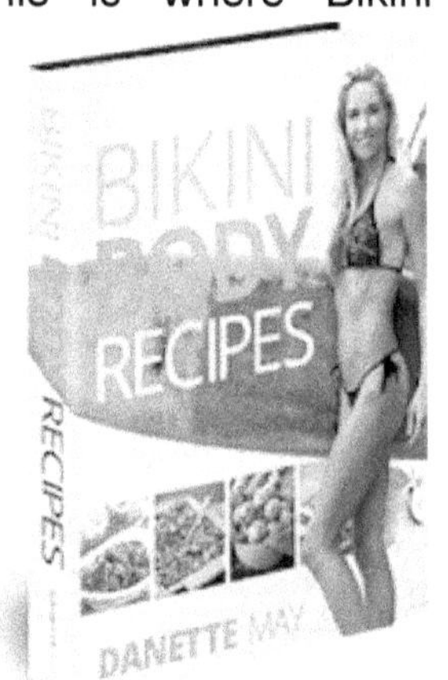

EAT MORE to LOSE MORE

Eat 6 times a day

Yes, you read it right – its 6 times a day. Not 3 times a day, but SIX times a day, every day!). This is what makes the Bikini Body method so different to those starvation diets where you deprive yourself and just stay hungry.

You should NEVER make yourself hungry - it sends all the wrong signals to your body. It takes just 10 minutes to whip up these delicious meals using only 5 ingredients.

Hair Bikers Diet Club

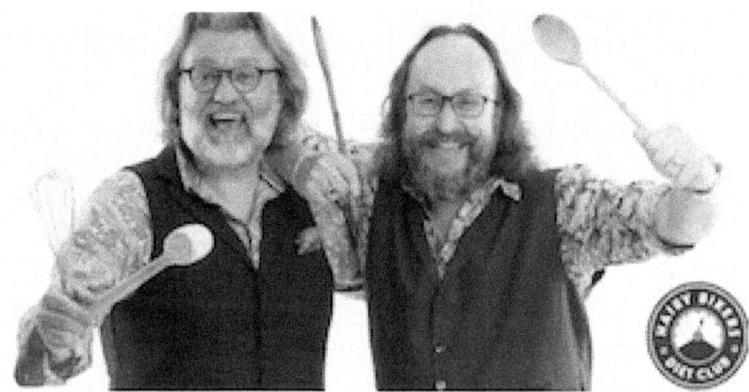

The Hairy Biker duo are **Si King**, and **Dave Myers**. They are two hairy-faced, and very down-to-earth cooks who share a love for hearty, wholesome food. They are well known all over the UK (and further beyond) from their BBC TV series *The Hairy Bikers*.

Both the bikers simply love food and they can't get enough of it. The problem is, after so many years of eating anything (and everything!) they wanted, they found that they were piling the pounds (and the stones) on. It began to affect their health.

In 2012 they realised they both faced a problem after Si became quite ill with type 2 diabetes and was pronounced morbidly obese facts; they decided to face the facts and got on the scales.

"Losing Weight saved my Life!"   Si King

They both set out to lose weight and decided to shared their weight loss journey with viewers to their TV show. Si and Dave lost 3 stone each in a short period of three months. They accomplished real weight loss just by making small changes and cutting back on their daily food portions.

Diets That Work

The Hairy Bikers also devised healthier versions of their favourite recipes. Dave and Si didn't really diet, they certainly didn't change their lives nor did they live on lettuce and water. All they did was indulge themselves, but in a healthier lifestyle, which meant eating good food and just a bit more exercise.

The Hairy Dieters book is chock full of all their favorite recipes, which just happen to also be healthy. When it was published it knocked the top selling Fifty Shades of Grey off its spot at the top of the UK bestseller chart.

"Health and happiness" is a subject that's very close to both Hairy Bikers and they have decided to share it with their viewers and fans all over the UK. They have now formed the Hairy Bikers Diet Club to help everyone else get fit and healthy and enjoy a great lifestyle.

Remember
It's all about good food not rabbit food.

A BLOKE'S GUIDE TO DIETING WITH CONFIDENCE

Here's a short extract from the

Hairy Bikers' Blog for Blokes.

"Back in the day when we were just lads, it was generally considered to be a bit 'unmanly' for geezers to keep careful watch what we ate. Us blokes were expected to tuck into giant steak sandwiches, in doorstep size bread of course, washed down with at least a couple of pints of beer.

Let's just take a few moments time out right now to salivate over that image: Steak, bread and beer . . . mmmm. Ah ! The memories!

We were definitely not expected to worry about things like carbs and calories and what the..."

Diets that Work

You can get instant access to the Blog, the videos, the recipes and all the other instruction and tips, just by joining our Hairy Bikers' Diet Club.

The *Hairy Bikers Diet Club* has several sections, one of which is bound to be ideally suited to YOU. There are special diets for women and for men; each have videos, help and advice, covering all meals and exercise and the knowledge and skills to create delicious meals for you and your family.

EAT GOOD FOOD NOT RABBIT FOOD!

- 210 Menu plans
- PLUS 400 Exercise programs
- Online diary to track calories
- Weekly weigh-ins
- Bags of motivation
- A buzzing community
- Recipes, tips, and lots more!

SLIM & SAVE with SI & DAVE

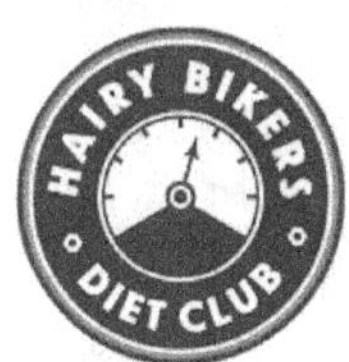

BodyWeight Burn

Eat carbs and enjoying favourite foods as you burn belly fat away - EVERY DAY! Anyone can sculpt their body to one that they deserve in just 21 minutes a day

> no matter your age

> no matter which gender

> no matter how fit you are

The Bodyweight Burn system features the BW3 Multiburn System. Its one that you can sculpt for yourself the body that you deserve in just 21 minutes a day. It doesn't matter how old you are or your fitness level.

You can continue enjoying your favourite foods while your metabolism burns away belly fat every day. Exercising too much can actually cause your body to store more fat, and you will learn by with the BodyWeight Burn system.

Adam Steer, who is also known as "The Bodyweight Coach"

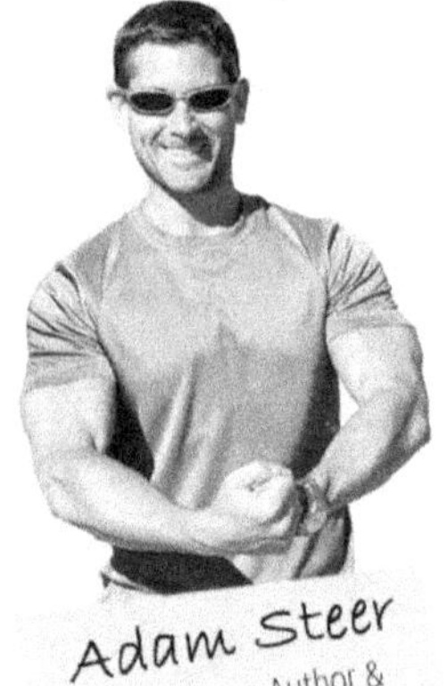

shares his methods, which have now proved to help clients get the bodies they deserve. And its all done without having to give up the foods they love. Nor do they have to spend hours on a treadmill or at the gym.

The entire Bodyweight Burn System can be quickly downloaded to any laptop or desktop computer, even to your tablet or phone so you can take it everywhere with you and lose the weight quicker. If you can spare 21 minutes a day, you can do it.

Diets that Work

Equipment-free Workouts!

The **BodyBurn System** teaches you how exercise can

1. Increase your Fat

2. Make you very ill,

3. KILL YOU !

There's a myth about how doing long workouts gets you results. Here's why that's just not true. Long and punishing workouts are proven to increase the stress hormones in your body, especially CORTISOL. In normal doses, cortisol is great because it helps the body to burn fat! In high doses however, such as those produced by long and stressful exercise, it forces the body into a 'protection mode'. The effect of this makes the body store more fat, and particularly around the stomach and on the hips.

The fat produced by high levels of the cortisol hormone turns into the stubborn fat that's almost impossible to lose, at least for as long as your cortisol remains at high levels. The biggest problem however is that the fat produced is of the kind that increases our risk of three terrible afflictions: diabetes, heart disease and cancer.

To lose weight you should NEVER workout for more than 30 minutes. 21 minutes gives you all the weight loss you need.

*   Burn a bit of belly fat every day

*   Experience more energy

*   Reduce aches, pains & injuries

*   Enjoy eating more carbs

*   Use your own bodyweight

*   With zero Equipment!

. Carbs After Dark

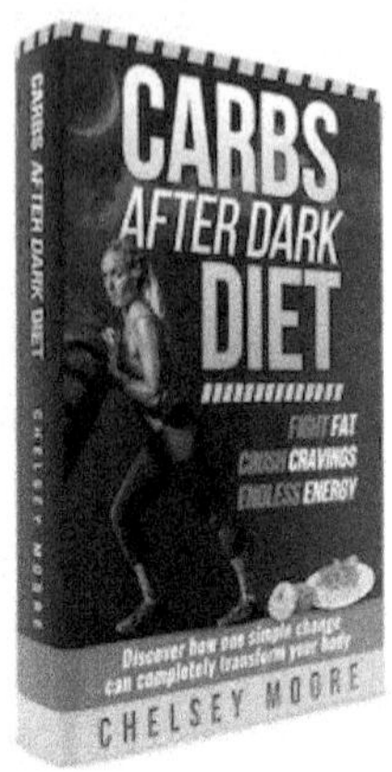

Carbs After Dark is the right course for you if you want to lose body weight fast you want to gain lean muscle you want more energy you want better performance you want to improve your social life.

Here's what's included

1. THE CARBS MANUAL

2. BONUS   Meal Ideas Guide

3. BONUS   The Workout Guide

4. BONUS   Protein Treats

Did you know that 'Nutrient Timing can strip YOUR body of all that unwanted excess fat with very little effort at all? Most people know that carbohydrate intake plays a crucial role in fat loss. The problem? Most people eliminate carbs all together. This is one of the worst things you can do. By eliminating carbs you slow down your metabolism, meaning you lack energy, and you get that unpleasant 'low carb brain' where you constantly feel groggy and moody.

  Chelsey Moore has been there and she says "Carbs aren't the problem - the way you're eating them is the problem."

Carbs After Dark is a great 'weight loss' regime devised by Chelsey and one which has been VERY successful for thousands of Americans who wanted to lose weight, and they did using this method.

Carbs After Dark makes losing fat so easy and pretty effortless because you don't have to cut out any particular food groups. In fact, you'll be surprised to learn how some of YOUR favorite foods can actually HELP you get rid of that stubborn fat that you have been trying for ages to burn off.

Diets that Work

The **Carbs After Dark** plan is very simple to follow; it can be customized to you and your schedule. Best of all, Carbs After Dark gets you results FAST! You'll start seeing and feeling changes after your first week! You'll be leaner, sleep better and have way more energy.

The Carbs After Dark plan will result in:

- Noticeable changes to your appearance in days!

- Enjoy carbs every day while burning fat.

- Turning your body into a fat burner

- Experiencing dieting freedom - no restrictions

- Having endless energy - no more crashes

You can try the **Carbs After Dark** programme RISK FREE! To protect you, there is a 60 day 'money back guarantee' and its all currently on offer at the low price of £9.95. You can pay with a card or Paypal from any country and the information and course is sent immediately.

Just a final note about Low Carb Diets from Chelsey. She says "Low Carb Diets are NOT for you. They can even be dangerous, because they do five bad things to you:

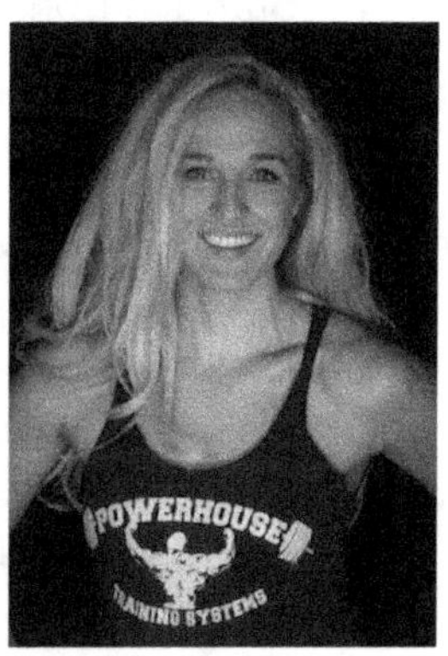

- slow your metabolism

- cause food cravings

- deplete energy levels

- cause mood swings

- mess with your hormones

please, don't even entertain a Low Carb diet. Listen to your body."

29 Day Flat Stomach

an unusual 10 minute a day trick
that can melt away a stone of belly fat.

Do you want a FLAT STOMACH? It can be done, in less than a month, and without spending a fortune on expensive gym equipment. Many women say their biggest and most stressful problem is that their husband thinks that they are too fat. Does it HURT that he thinks you are, like most wives, just a little too fat?

LEPTIN RESISTANCE

Maybe you are the victim of a little known hormonal disorder that is making your belly too fat? Try this 3 second test:

1. Stand in front of a long mirror

2. Place both hands on your belly

3. GRAB

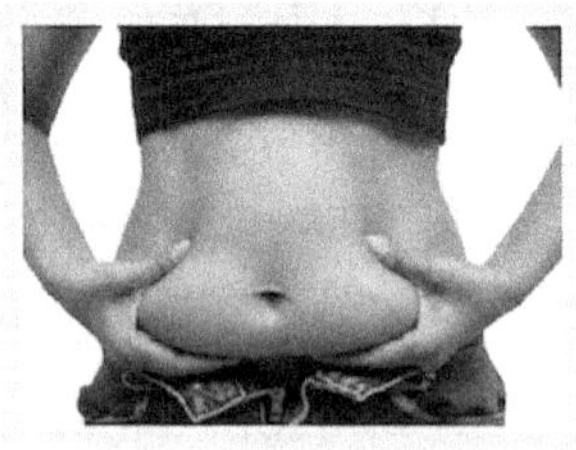

If you have a handful of fat in each hand, you're 'Leptin Resistant' And you can finally stop feeling guilty and depressed about your weight as you simply have a condition that was never diagnosed and properly treated. The good news is that YOU can turn OFF your Leptin Resistance.

Derek Wahler is a trainer known as the Weight Whisperer. Derek has a reputation of taking on the most difficult women and men who haven't been able to lose weight for years and transform their bodies in just minutes right in their own living room. Because his methods are so short and simple, it's possible to see results after just a few day!

The Weight Whisperer spotted the one serious problem that was sabotaging results - **Too much strenuous exercise!**

Diets that Work

This leads to uncontrollable inflammation in the belly and that makes it impossible to burn belly fat.

HYPERTENSION

The other problem the Weight Whisperer addresses is **HYPERTENSION**. This is seriously raised Blood Pressure and Heart Hypertension, if undetected and ignored, can cause silent heart failure <u>WITHOUT WARNING.</u>

Here is what the NHS says:

> *High blood pressure, or hypertension, rarely has noticeable symptoms. But if untreated, it increases your risk of serious problems such as heart attacks and strokes.*
>
> *More than one in four adults in the UK have high blood pressure, although many don't realise it.*
>
> *The only way to find out if your blood pressure is high is to have your blood pressure checked.*

(I have a blood pressure monitor and it every day, as it gives a sure indication of anything going wrong, before it does. For £50 it's a small investment to make sure this important indication is spotted early enough to do something about it and save your life!)

Pockets of fat in overweight people put EXTREME PRESSURE on the lungs, arteries, and are a cause of Heart Hypertension. This is the number one cause of death associated with high blood pressure and eventually leads to heart failure.

ACT TODAY and perhaps you will save your own life! You don't need expensive equipment and you can do this in your own home, at work, or in fact ANYwhere! The **29 Day Flat Stomach** system costs only £15 – details are on a separate page on our web site.

Eat Stop Eat

This is dieting for ANYONE

- **Too Old?**

- **Too Fat?**

- **Too Sick?**

- **No Time?**

- **No Will Power**?

Eat Stop Eat is a diet that really works and it works IMMEDIATELY We tried it and saw very quick results. The 'Eat Stop eat' book is easy to follow and it's crammed with proven information and tips to help you lose POUNDS in a very short time, and without cutting out your favourite foods.

As part of Eat Stop Eat, author Brad Pilon outlines a method which does help shed pounds.

This is a new theory of dieting. It enables you to can take control of your weight, and how you feel, and doesn't use faddish starvation regimes, exercise routines or other ideas that are hard to follow.

Simply eat your normal evening meal tonight. Straight afterwards, start using the simple instructions in *Eat Stop Eat* on page 116.   Tomorrow night after your evening meal, answer these questions:

- Do you feel lighter?

- Is there more bounce in your step?

- Your system feel cleaner & healthier?

- Are feel more clear headed and alert?

The very next morning, weigh yourself. Are you 1-3 lbs lighter? Wait one more week and weigh yourself again, at the

Diets that Work

same time of day. Do you see that your weight has dropped another 3-5 pounds?

By now you should also be feeling that each time you use the *Eat Stop Eat* protocol it just gets easier and you feel less and less hungry. Hunger will lose almost all its grip on you and your old cravings should all but disappear!

In a month's time, put on the same clothes you're wearing today and look in the mirror. The Eat Stop Eat diet asks:

- Are your clothes hanging off you?

- Is your face looking leaner?

- Do you feel younger, brighter?

- Have you got more energy?

- Have you lost that "brain fog"

The brain fog is quite common that we get used to, and its what is usually holding us down. It's easy to get excited that you now have no forbidden foods.

I love it when I can reward myself with all my favorite food. Social eating for me is a celebration again and no longer a burden.

Diets That Work

Frequently Asked Questions

Q: Can I lose fat and gain muscle ?

Yes! *Eat Stop Eat* outlines exactly how you can build muscle while simultaneously losing body fat. Read the chapter 'Fasting and your muscle mass' for more information.

Q: Is it OK for women to miss meals?

A: The *Eat Stop Eat* style of eating has helped thousands of women lose weight. There is an entire chapter in Eat Stop Eat devoted to helping women get the absolute best results possible from Eat Stop Eat, you can check out the chapter 'Fasting for women' for more information.

Q: Does it maintain your current weight?

A: Absolutely! *Eat Stop Eat* gives you a simple way to lose weight, and to maintain your weight. Timing is the trick. If you want to not only lose weight, but keep it off, there is a special chapter covering just that.

Q: Any guarantee I will lose weight?

A: No, no-one can do that. *Eat Stop Eat* does not have a weight loss guarantee and nor does any other diet. If a diet claims to do that then beware, as its probably scamming you. A Weight Loss program needs you to eat less and exercise more. *Eat Stop Eat* is a book outlining all the principles you need to be very successful at losing weight and keeping it off. It's up to YOU however to actually put all the principles into action. *Eat Stop Eat* can only help YOU make that happen.

DIET BOOKS

There are hundreds of books about diet and nutrition. There are perhaps even tens of thousands of books if one includes those titles which are now 'out of print' and no longer easily obtainable! We have found very few diet books that credibly describe diets that we could be certain actually DO work.

This section discusses those diet books that we can recommend and are relevant to diets discussed on other pages on the Diets That Work site.

Be Skinny Fast   by Nolan Smith

Nolan Smiths well known diet book has the tag line: "The Diet that Works motivates and instructs."

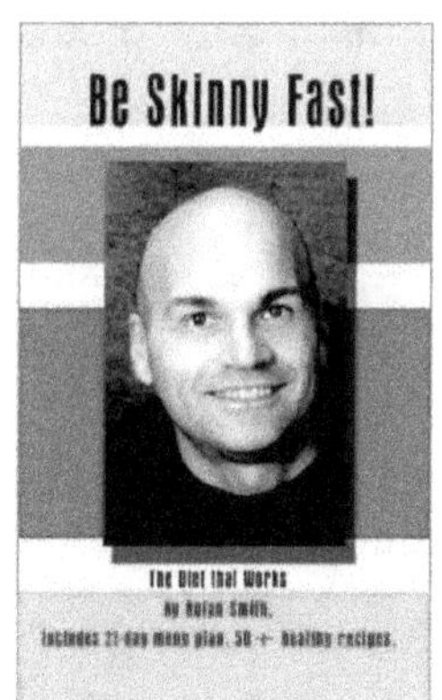

Be Skinny Fast includes a lot of recipes to replace bread, sugars and fried foods, which Nolan advises you drop from your diet. His method works, although it does take some working at. Some will say that if you are "skinny" this is not healthy, but if you need a diet that will drop the pounds then this is a good bet. Its 224 pages long and is a paperback, published in 2002.

One of the book's reviewers (Don Walker) comments that they lost 20 pounds by sticking to the diet proposed by Nolan. They virtually eliminated sugar from their diet and recommended the book, saying that he felt more vibrant and energetic with Nolan's plan.

You can get the book via a link on our web site.

Vitamins & Minerals

How to get the nutrients your body needs

by Sarah Rose

This is a book full of the practical advice about the many and various vitamins and minerals that your body needs, and so you can understand what each of them does. The book explains why you needs each one and when is the optimum time to take them.

Sarah's book also explains how the nutritional needs of our bodies can be expected to change at all stages throughout our lives and it also describes the various types of supplements that are available to supplement our diet.

With 300 colourful pages, this book makes choosing a healthy lifestyle easy and enjoyable and helps you to assess your specific needs and find out how to tailor your diet and lifestyle to suit these.

(This book can be notoriously hard to find – we have links to it on the BOOKS page on the web site.)

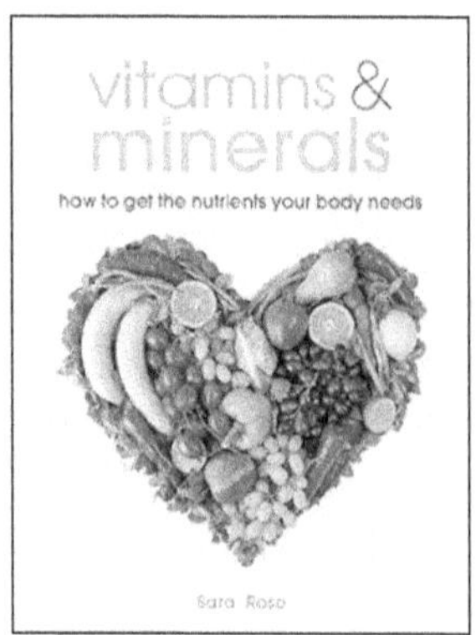

BODY SCULPTING for men and women

Although still only available as Kindles, these books are billed as the "Deluxe Platinum editions, bigger and better!" This means more work-outs, more on nutrition and more exercise for anyone wanting a total makeover of their physique.

At 400 pages, these are very comprehensive books and cover a 21 day express workout with many time-saving exercises. They also include lots of tips and helpful information to keep up your motivation and to help you achieve your desired fitness goals.

The regime for women seems less demanding; for example, it has a 14 day express Sculpting Workshop to follow which is intended to sculpt, slim and strengthen particular contours of women's bodies. This includes toned arms, flat abs, lean legs, tight buns and the curves all in the places you would expect.

The books are written by James Villepigue who has over twenty years experience in the health and fitness industry. He has appeared in many magazine articles and TV programmes and trains top athletes and artists.

Kindles can be read on almost any equipment with a screen, including iPads and other tablets, and both lap-top and full sized computers. To get more details of the books, which are available as separate editions for men or for women see the details on our web site.

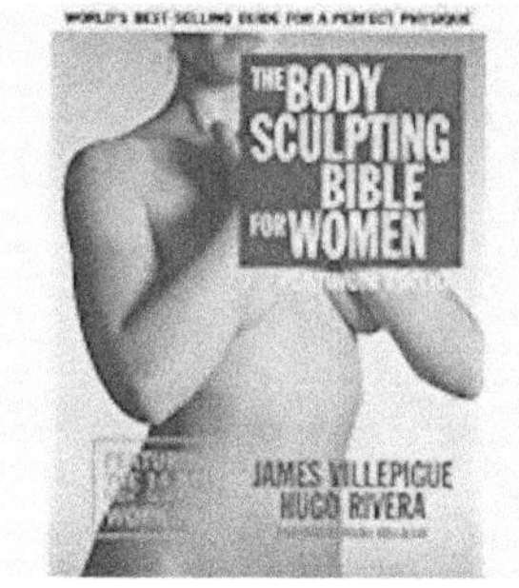

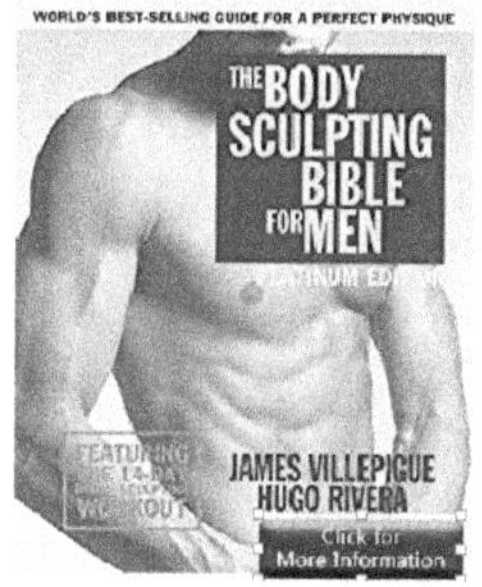

Diets That Work

Glycaemic Load and its effect on diet

GL stands for Glycaemic Load. It's a unit of measurement that tells you exactly what a particular food will do to your blood sugar.

Foods with the highest Glycaemic Load levels have a much greater effect on your blood sugar, which isn't at all wanted. It's important to know what those foods are.

On the other hand, those foods with a low GL will more easily encourage the body to burn fat. That is the ideal situation in reducing weight.

 Keeping the levels of blood sugar and the balance between them is the key concept at the core of the low GL Diet. Once that is achieved then sustainable weight loss will follow.

The GL Diet has often been described as "the perfect way to lose weight, gain energy and improve your overall health."

Patrick Holford's revolutionary **Low GL Diet** is based on achieving a good balance of your blood sugars and is one of the safest and most effective ways to lose weight. A truly effective, easy-to-follow diet that will not only help you lose weight and put an end to cravings, but also boost your energy and improve your health

Diets that Work

Low GL Diet Cookbook

By Patrick Holford, BSc, DipON, FBANT

The Low-GL Diet Cookbook is perfect for everyone who wants to lose weight quickly, yet still enjoy great-tasting food. Featured in the book are a very wide range of recipes, but ones that will not raise your blood sugar too quickly leading to your body having a much lower glyceamic load, or GL.

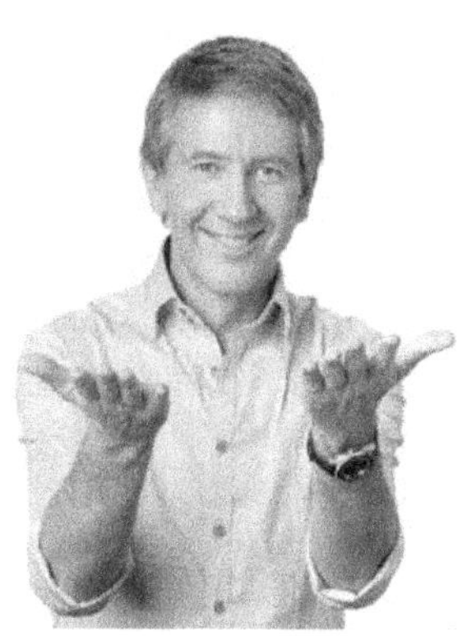

Based on the latest research, top nutritionist Patrick Holford explains that by having no more than 40 GLs a day and eating protein with carbohydrate, you can not only lose weight quickly and permanently but also improve your health and feel truly energised.

The book is packed with delicious tried-and-tested recipes that are both easy to follow and simple to prepare. The GL of each recipe is clearly calculated for you, so it's easy to stick to your daily limit, and with menu plans and recipes for both weight-loss and maintenance,

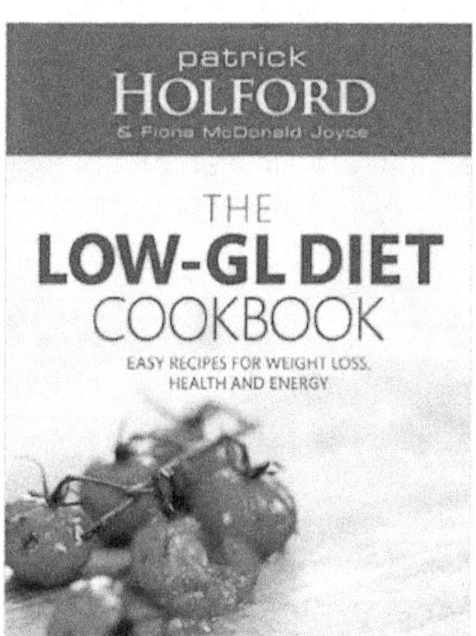

If you are looking for a good way to beat cravings and lose excess body weight permanently, then the Low GL Diet Cookbook is likely to be a good investment. There are links on the web site to find this book of delicious recipes.

Endurance Training Diet Cookbook

Jesse's unique has his own special unique approach to nutrition. In it he combines an engineer's mind-set with his own extensive athletic experience. Jesse researched and organized every aspect of training and nutrition that the endurance athlete needs to improve their daily eating and drinking choices. The result is a very detailed programme that has tremendous effect on one's metabolism and at the same time easy to follow.

Jesse's detailed approach to fueling (eating and drinking, both are very important) that he shares in his book, can change your life if you are an athlete and especially a runner.

Author Jesse Kropelnicki is a veteran professional triathlon coach and the founder of QT2 Systems brand of endurance sports preparation businesses. His roster of clients includes many champions and national team athletes.

"The Endurance Training Diet & Cookbook" has a mass of knowledge that athletes of whatever their level or skill set can learn from. This is an ideal mixture of education, knowledge, tips, and easy-to-make recipes. Athletes are always seeking healthy recipes that are simple to prepare, nutrient rich and they all taste good, too! Many of them can be found in this book.

Exercise Equipment

The beauty of many of the diets we found that worked best were those that did not require a lot of equipment. Those that involved any exercise at all relied on everyday items as 'props'.

There is a wide range of exercise and fitness equipment on the market now, although it can be intimidating visiting the showrooms where such items are on display. Over zealous salesmen (and they are always men, rarely are women allowed onto the shop floor to sell fitness equipment!) will pounce, with their 'oh so superior' attitude and dismissive air.

You won't find any of that behaviour at DKN's on line service. We recommend DKN machinery for several reasons. It's all ergonomically designed to provide comfort in use whilst looking great in the home. If you are looking to keep healthy and fit now and for many years to come, then DKN have the right exercise kit for you. By going right to the supplier you will get the best possible deal, the right kit for your needs, and their after service is nothing short of perfect.

Take a look at DKN's web site, which has every imaginable contraption or piece of equipment you will need for safe and comfortable exercise.

ACCESSORIES

DKN are not just THE place to go to for the major items of equipment, but they stock a wide variety of fitness accessories too.

Gym balls, aerobic setups, exercise mats, hand-grips of all types, motion cradles and even scales and pedometers. DKN make or distribute almost every imaginable piece of equipment you may need to follow a strict exercise regime.

Diets That Work

M500 Incline Trainer

This machine has all the benefits you might expect of a treadmill but with intensified performance. It can be inclined to up to 40%, so reproduces the most arduous slopes anyone could be expected to tackle in training.

Combining the action of a cross trainer, a fully-fledged step machine and a top rated treadmill all in one efficient piece of home workout kit. Owners of this machine can enjoy safe, low-impact cardio sessions thanks to the 40 variable levels of Power Incline up to a top speed of 7.5mph (12kph).

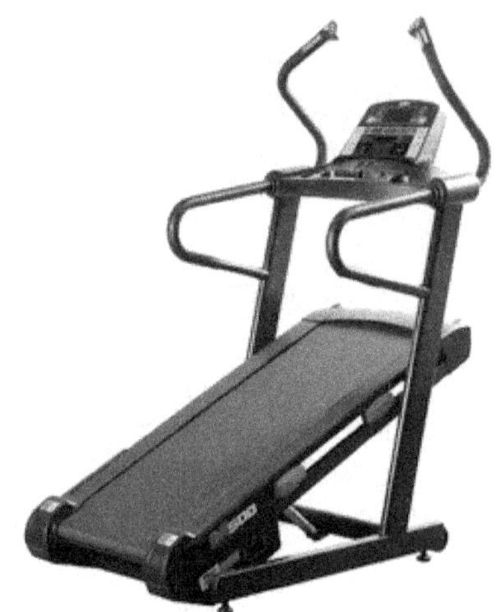

You will be able to burn up more calories and get excellent muscle definition on this machine, which is a top quality trainer that works muscles through a wider range of motion compared to other fitness machines.

The M500 Incline Trainer also boasts the Progressive Shock Absorbing system which reduces impacts giving its user a far more comfortable and safer exercising. Incline and speed can be selected using the One Touch Control buttons and you have easy access to the nine workout programmes, so you can vary the challenges every day of the week.

You can measure heart rate through the hand pulse sensors, or via a wireless receiver and an optional chest belt. It's easy to follow your progress on the hi-contrast blue backlit LCD console and enjoy the additions of speakers, an mp3 audio port and a cooling fan to make your workout experience even more of a pleasure. You watch the calories used and check on your progress.

The Incline Trainer comes with a full 12 month Warranty and is delivered FREE – check it out on our equipment page on the web site.

Studio 9000 Multi Gym

The DKN Studio 9000 Multi Gym is a versatile home workstation designed to help you develop all areas of your body. This Multi Gym enables you to perform many exercises such as the chest press, shoulder press, low pulley row, bicep curls, pull downs, leg extensions and inner / outer leg kicks.

Moreover, the gym bench can also be upgraded with an optional leg press to help you strengthen the quads. Thanks to the workout bench's adjustable upholstery and frame the sessions with the machine become safer as well as more comfortable and precise. This useful piece of gym equipment comes complete with a lat bar, a short bar and an ankle strap.

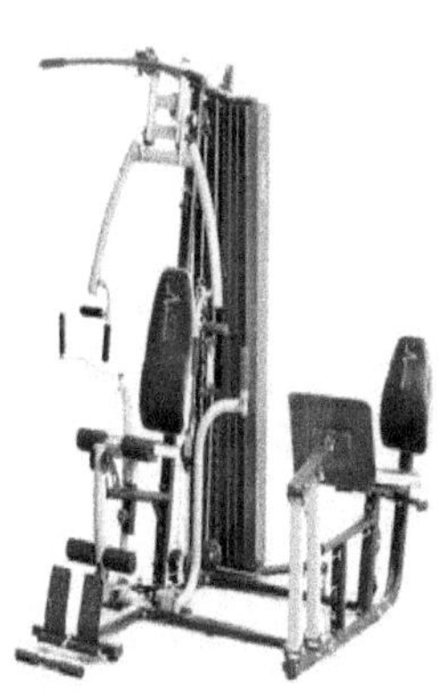

Over 20 exercises are possible (crunch, low pulley row, front and lateral shoulder raise, lat pull down, inner and outer leg kick, seated shoulder press, abdominal leg raise, narrow-grip pull down, standing biceps curl and standing leg curl, butterfly and more).

Full details of the MultiGym can be found on the Equipment pages of our web site.

AM 5i Ergo Exercise Bike

The console of the DKN AM-5i ergo exercise bike enables the user to choose from twelve professionally designed programmes, use heart rate control zone and Watt training, as well as store individual data for personal workout information.

This is ideal for counting the calories as they burn away all kinds of weight loss. See full details of the AM 5i Ergo on our web site along with several other models – there is likely to be one ideally suited to your particular requirements. All models qualify for free delivery in the UK.

Elliptical Cross Trainer

The DKN XC-140i elliptical cross trainer has a function-rich console with 2-colour backlit LCD display. That gives constant feedback on your important workout data such as time, speed, distance, calories, watts and heart rate. Four user profiles can store age, gender, weight and height info and offer a choice of workout programmes. Included are 12 pre-set (4 beginner, 4 advanced, 4 performance) and one manual programme.

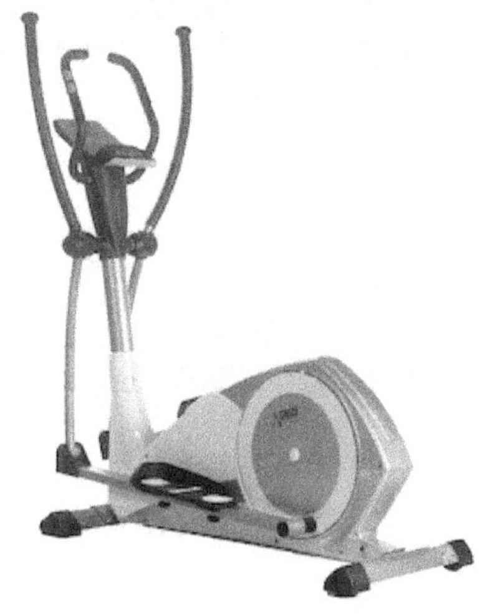

This cross trainer has pulse grip sensors to monitor heart rate and a wireless receiver for more accurate monitoring. The DKN XC-140i is compatible with *iPad* and most recent Android tablets.

After having completed your workout you have the possibility to save the crucial statistics of training such as date, duration and the total amount of calories burned can be stored.

The DKN Motion application lets you 'explore' many iconic routes from all around the world, with built-in *iRoutes*. The Elliptical Cross Trainer's resistance changes to match elevations that would be encountered, which makes it more realistic. Progress can be followed with a moving pointer on the map of the route.

Also included XC-140i Cross Trainer is the *iWorld* application (a FREE App - details at the *iTunes* Store). With this App you can explore any place on the globe, plan your own routes and follow a route online using *Streetview*.

Diets That Work

A Note from the Author

Thank you for reading the book this far, we hope you enjoyed it and that it has fired you up with more enthusiasm for losing weight. You WILL feel much better. Just imagine, all your old clothes fitting you perfectly once again.

Most of the information in this book is taken from our web site, where you can find even more details. The site is updated often. If we haven't covered a topic in which you are interested, it's likely to be on there somewhere. If you cant find it, send me an email and either I, or one of my team, will be delighted to try and help.

You can email me at *Anne@dietsthatwork.co.uk.*

There is also a Kindle edition of the book available on Amazon. It includes all the hyperlinks, so you can navigate to further information more easily.

Anne Alexander

Anne Alexander